A Guide to Anger Management

Hartley is a writer and personal development coach specializing
le skills and communication. She has considerable experience
g on these topics and of presenting workshops and courses
ts of interpersonal communication and behaviour. As well as
ting to national newspapers and women's and general-interest
les, Mary has broadcast on national and local radio programmes
s such as managing anger and coping with stress, and has acted
ultant for the BBC Learning Zone. Her books *The Good Stress Guide*,
ng *Anger at Work*, *Stress at Work*, *The Assertiveness Handbook*, *The
man's Handbook* and *How to Listen so that People Talk* are all pub-
y Sheldon Press.

Overcoming Common Problems Series

Selected titles

A full list of titles is available from Sheldon Press,
36 Causton Street, London SW1P 4ST and on our website at
www.sheldonpress.co.uk

Overcoming Common Problems Series

Overcoming Common Problems Series

Overcoming Common Problems

A Guide to Anger Management

MARY HARTLEY

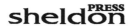
sheldon PRESS

First published in Great Britain in 2009

Sheldon Press
36 Causton Street
London SW1P 4ST

The author and publisher have made every effort to ensure that the
external website and email addresses included in this book are correct and
up to date at the time of going to press. The author and publisher are not
responsible for the content, quality or continuing accessibility of the sites.

British Library Cataloguing-in-Publication Data
A catalogue record for this book is available from the British Library

ISBN 978-1-84709-072-0

1 3 5 7 9 10 8 6 4 2

Typeset by Fakenham Photosetting Ltd, Fakenham, Norfolk
Printed in Great Britain by Ashford Colour Press

Produced on paper from sustainable forests

Contents

1

Women in an angry society

Anger can be a frightening emotion. We often associate it with verbal and physical violence, with shouting, screaming, throwing things, hitting, lashing out. Our personal experiences of everyday life and the media coverage of angry and violent incidents paint a picture of a society consumed by uncontrollable anger and rage. It seems that the strains and pressures of contemporary life are resulting in many of us becoming more impatient and intolerant, responding angrily to even minor and commonplace frustrations and annoyances.

The Civil Aviation Authority has reported a 400 per cent increase in air rage incidents between 1997 and 2000. The annual Social Trends Survey shows that complaints about loud music, barking dogs and similar disturbances have increased five-fold in the last twenty years. The British Association for Anger Management reports that the UK has the dubious distinction of being the second-worst country in the world for road rage, with more than 80 per cent of drivers admitting to having been involved in such incidents. Even the office is not exempt from violent eruptions of anger, with 65 per cent of office workers admitting to losing their tempers to the extent of throwing objects at their computer screens and screaming abuse at colleagues.

The way that we attach the word 'rage' to the cause or context of violent eruptions of anger – road rage, air rage, computer rage, phone rage, to name but a few – indicates the extent to which such incidents occur, but also has the effect of suggesting that somehow 'rage' incidents are an unavoidable and inescapable part of life. Constant eruptions of anger, it seems, are the inevitable consequence of living at a pace and speed that were unimaginable a short time ago. It is only to be expected that so many of us are unable to respond in any other way to the pressures of contemporary life.

1

However, rage is not inevitable, nor is it the only way of responding. There are better ways of dealing with angry feelings. Anger is a powerful, valuable emotion. Anger tells us when we feel hurt or abused or threatened, and spurs us to take action to protect ourselves. It is an instinctive, natural emotion which enables us to deal with danger. Healthy anger is based on sound and accurate appraisals of situations, and is expressed with appropriate words and actions and in a suitable context. This is the most positive way of handling anger, one which enables us to channel our emotions safely and constructively and is likely to lead to an outcome in which feelings are expressed openly and no one is physically or mentally damaged. If we all managed our angry feelings in this way, anger wouldn't be a problem for individuals or for society. Disputes and conflicts, clashes of opinion and interests and feelings of hurt and frustration would be dealt with in a civilized and controlled fashion, and we would develop greater understanding of and tolerance for each other. We would be safer and happier.

Women and anger

It is a common idea that men are angrier than women, a view possibly shaped by the perception that men's anger is often physical and highly visible. Images of men fighting and behaving aggressively are commonplace and do not cause the kind of reaction which greets images of women acting in this way. Women's anger is often dismissed or trivialized as hysteria. Sometimes it is demonized, as if there is something unnatural about women experiencing such an emotion. Sometimes it is regarded as just a hormone-driven mood, something not to be taken seriously. Derogatory terms such as 'bitch' and 'nag' are directed against women who express angry feelings. Small wonder, then, that women's anger is often invisible, sometimes even to themselves.

In fact, women experience angry feelings just as often as men do, if not more so. The difference is that women manage these feelings differently, often shying away from outright expressions of hostility and rage. There are social and historical explanations for this. For generations in the past, women were not encouraged to give voice to their feelings or to display any 'unpleasant' emotions. They would bottle up and repress angry and uncomfortable feelings rather than reveal them openly, a choice which women often continue to make nowadays. Many women are uncomfortable with expressing anger, and are frightened of the power it unleashes. We see anger as something to be ashamed of, as a negative emotion which needs to be hidden and stifled. Women are seen by others and by ourselves as nurturers and caregivers, and so we feel we cannot be angry with people without undermining our vital roles. So we smile instead of speaking sharply, swallow hurt and resentment rather than let it show, and smooth things over rather than stir up discord and arguments.

This might seem like a good way of achieving a peaceful existence. But choosing to bury feelings of anger is in the end unproductive and, as we will see, can be damaging to our health as well as to our relationships.

However, some recent studies have shown that women are looking for positive ways of handling their anger. The British Association of Anger Management reports an increase in the numbers of women attending its anger management courses. Women are learning to acknowledge their anger and to channel their feelings of frustration into creating change in their lives, and are in a good position to do so. It is the traditionally 'female' strengths which show the way to effective anger management. The so-called 'soft skills' of communication, negotiation and problem-solving are powerful tools in the fight against being overwhelmed by anger and frustration. Other strategies for coping with upset and angry feelings include approaches that women tend to be used to and good at, such as talking things over with a friend, or looking for solutions rather than conflict. We can build on our strengths and learn to use anger to bring about improvements in our lives and our relationships. Anger, used positively and effectively, can highlight problems and imbalances in relationships; it can help to right wrongs; it can lead to self-knowledge, honesty and mutual respect.

Exercise 1.1: Your ideas about anger

Use this list to help you to identify your attitude to expressions of anger.

	Strongly agree	Agree	Disagree
It's not nice for women to show anger.	☐	☐	☐
I find it difficult to express myself when I'm angry and upset.	☐	☐	☐
When I'm angry, I'm scared of losing control.	☐	☐	☐
I don't like upsetting people.	☐	☐	☐
I'm afraid of creating a bad atmosphere.	☐	☐	☐
Showing anger is a sign of weakness.	☐	☐	☐
People will turn against me if I'm angry with them.	☐	☐	☐
It's always better to laugh something off, even if it has made you angry.	☐	☐	☐
I like to be the one to keep the peace.	☐	☐	☐
If I'm angry with people they will think I don't like/love them.	☐	☐	☐
There's no point in getting angry.	☐	☐	☐
I'd rather get my own back on someone than tell them how I'm feeling.	☐	☐	☐
When I'm angry, I take it out on someone else.	☐	☐	☐
I think it's always better to grit your teeth and bear it.	☐	☐	☐
I believe in always turning the other cheek.	☐	☐	☐
Being angry is the only way to get people to listen to me.	☐	☐	☐
I'd rather suffer in silence than cause a fuss.	☐	☐	☐
I show my anger by dropping hints.	☐	☐	☐
When I'm angry I go into silent mode.	☐	☐	☐
When I'm angry I sulk until someone asks me what's wrong.	☐	☐	☐

If you strongly agree with one or more of the above statements, you are probably not managing your anger effectively. Consciously or unconsciously, you behave in ways which deny, repress or misdirect your feelings. You may have drifted into or inherited unhelpful ways of handling anger. However, even though your pattern of response may be well established, you can learn to break it and develop different strategies to help you to regulate and channel anger and put it to positive uses.

Make positive use of your 'female' qualities

Studies suggest that certain ways of communicating are characteristically female. Some of these ways of behaving could prevent you from expressing your anger effectively if you let their negative qualities hold sway. Instead, work to the strengths of these characteristics, and allow their positive aspects to support your communication.

It's a female thing ...

Being indirect

- Examples: dropping hints; understating or skirting round the issue; speaking to someone other than the person involved hoping that the message will be passed on; sulking; the silent treatment.
- Drawbacks: if you don't make your point clearly and unmistakeably, there is every chance that the other person will miss what you are trying to say. Your message might be missed entirely, or its importance might not be recognized.
- Strengths: your innate tactfulness can help you to address the issue without diminishing or attacking the other person. You can learn to be honest without being brutally so.

Avoiding conflict and confrontation

- Examples: putting up with something that really annoys you to avoid an argument; saying that nothing is wrong when you are seething inside.
- Drawbacks: if you do not face up to an issue, you are likely to suffer the negative effects of bottling up your feelings. The problem will not go away and will not be solved.
- Strengths: you can learn how to channel your dislike of aggression into assertive communication. You can discover ways in which conflict can be handled constructively. The way in which you deal with conflict can demonstrate to others how it can be done, so that you become a role model for the people you live and work with.

Being collaborative and co-operative

- Examples: being willing to concede on issues; looking for solutions to problems.
- Drawbacks: you might underplay your own feelings, or not be clear enough about what you want or where you stand on a matter.
- Strengths: the ability to work with people rather than against them is a vital part of managing anger. You can learn how to express your feelings clearly and you can develop skills of negotiation.

Wanting approval and to be liked

- Examples: not showing anger because you think other people will disapprove; thinking that revealing angry feelings will cause others to reject you.
- Drawbacks: your fear of losing people's approval or affection prevents you from communicating honestly. This could mean that your relationships suffer from lack of honest communication.
- Strengths: the fact that people matter to you means that you act with consideration for others' feelings. You can build your self-esteem and come to recognize that telling people when you are hurt or frustrated by their behaviour need not damage your relationship with them.

How anger affects your life

Anger is an uncomfortable emotion, and when we are in its thrall rather than managing it constructively the quality of our lives and our relationships is undermined.

We experience being angry in different ways. Some of us realize that our lives are marked by outbursts of rage, by tempers being frequently lost, by shouting matches with partners and children. Conversations are punctuated by the sounds of slamming doors and people storming out. Others suffer the quiet, insidious effects of anger that is held in, unable or too scared to speak openly about how they are feeling.

Steer clear of Tracey

Tracey finds her drive to work very stressful. The journey is made longer and more tedious by permanent road works which slow everything down and clog up the traffic. She gets very wound up and beeps her horn impatiently. She scowls at anyone who tries to change lanes in an awkward place, and shifts position to stop them getting in. By the time she gets to work she is fuming with rage, and it takes a good half hour for her to calm down.

Things aren't great at home either. Tracey can feel herself building up for a row with her mother, who has twice recently let her down over child-minding arrangements. Also niggling away at the back of her mind is the forthcoming parents' evening at her children's school, when she will be tackling Adam's teacher about an unfair comment in his homework journal. Just thinking about it makes her feel angry.

Tracey feels on edge all the time, so that even the slightest thing can make her fly into a rage. Her family, friends and work colleagues sense that she is always in a bad mood these days and tread warily around her, not wanting to spark any trouble.

Lisa won't make a fuss

Lisa hates the idea of confrontation, and prefers to keep quiet about things that annoy her rather than risk an argument. She knows that people take advantage of her easy-going nature. Because she is known not to drink a lot, everyone assumes that she will always be happy to be the designated driver when they go out; because she never queries anything she is asked to do at work, all the unpleasant or tedious tasks get dumped on her; because she never pushes her own point of view, her suggestions about what DVD to watch or what kind of take-away to get are generally ignored in favour of others' preferences.

No one knows that Lisa feels angry about being put upon all the time because she never reveals what is going on inside her. However, her feelings build up inside her so that sometimes she feels as if she is going to explode with pent-up rage. She feels tense and she constantly blames herself for not being stronger. Lisa's low self-esteem and lack of control over her life make her shrink down inside herself, but she continues to smile and agree with people and swallow her resentment.

The cost of mismanaged anger

If anger is not handled well, it can take its toll on all areas of your life.

Exercise 1.2: How angry feelings get in the way

Think about the ways in which angry feelings are getting in the way of your ability to deal with situations and to maintain and develop positive relationships.

At home

1 _____

2 _____

3 _____

At work

1 _____

2 _____

3 _____

Social life

1 _____

2 _____

3 _____

Now think about what will be changed for the better by dealing positively with feelings of hurt and anger.

You could focus on:

- how you will feel better physically;
- how your relationships will be improved;
- how you will feel about yourself;
- how your abilities to think clearly will be improved.

Add your own ideas:

	Area of my life	*What will be improved*
1		
2		
3		
4		
5		
6		

Skills to help

You can develop the skills that are needed to build on your strengths and use your personal attributes and qualities to deepen your understanding of your feelings of anger, rage, annoyance, frustration. Rather than let these feelings damage and limit your life, you can learn to accept them and channel them in directions that will benefit all aspects of your life.

The skills of managing anger effectively are based on the ability to observe and understand yourself and others; to be honest with yourself and others; to express your feelings clearly and appropriately to the right person; to express anger for the right reasons. Learning to do this is a challenging path to take, but may prove to be not only life-enhancing, but life-saving as well.

2

The nature of anger

Anger is a powerful and important emotion. It's our hard-wired response when we feel threatened in some way, a response designed to galvanize us into protecting ourselves and our property. When we perceive a threat to our well-being, or that our needs aren't being met, our body kicks into action to enable us to do something about the threat.

Our anger is aroused when, among other circumstances:

- We feel attacked or threatened.
- We feel put down or devalued.
- We feel that our person or property is at risk.
- We feel that someone or something is preventing us from getting what we want.
- We feel helpless.
- We feel that our principles and values are under attack.
- We feel humiliated.
- We feel exploited.

You may have ideas of your own to add to this list:

_____

_____

_____

How anger functions healthily

When something happens to cause us to get angry, our bodies adapt to help us deal with the threat. Our physical response to anger is automatic, as our bodies become aroused for action. A normal and healthy process is triggered, one which is designed to give us the strength to take the physical action that is required for self-protection. This reaction is sometimes referred to as the 'fight or flight' response – we are ready to fight back and attack the aggressor, or we are ready to run for our lives.

Think about the last time you were furious about something or with someone, a time when you felt that your person was attacked or threatened. It is likely that your heart started thumping, you went very red or you went very white, you spoke more loudly than usual, and your muscles became tense and tight.

These reactions were caused by the physical changes brought about as your nervous system utilized your body's resources to send help where it was needed. The release of adrenalin caused your arteries to constrict and your blood pressure to rise as blood was diverted to your heart and muscles, to give you strength to deal with the crisis. Your digestive system shut down (you may have noticed how in these circumstances your mouth goes dry and you lose your appetite) and your breathing increased to stimulate the amount of oxygen in your blood. Your body was on all systems go, ready to take action. Your mind was in gear as well, and you felt clear and confident about your ability to deal with the threat. You took whatever behaviour was appropriate.

When the incident was over, your body returned to normal. You calmed down, your breathing slowed, your muscles relaxed, and maybe you then felt like having a cup of tea or coffee. The danger or threat receded, and your body resumed its usual functions, replenishing its resources to be ready for the next time.

What happens when the process doesn't work

Being angry all the time

This protective process works when both its stages take place. The trouble is that if you're always or very frequently angry, the second part of the process doesn't happen. Being angry continues to make enormous demands on your body. You are on edge and punchy all the time, and your body is continually being fired up for action. It never has a chance to calm down, and is constantly teeming with stress hormones. This makes you vulnerable to a number of ailments, just some of which are:

- heart disease and strokes, caused by high blood pressure, elevated cholesterol levels and constricted blood vessels;
- digestive disorders, caused by the presence of acid;
- aches and pains, caused by tense muscles;
- exhaustion, caused by using up your store of energy through increased metabolic rate;
- kidney damage, caused by high blood pressure.

Being unable to express your anger

Not everyone will have responded in quite the way described. We all react in different ways. Some people feel invigorated and energized by their anger, others feel scared by its power and helpless to alter its course. It may be that feeling anger causes you to think less of yourself; maybe you see anger as something to be ashamed of, something 'nice' women don't feel towards the people in their lives and families. Perhaps experiencing other people's anger has caused you to fear its effect. You may in this case go into frozen mode, unable to move a muscle to do anything about the situation. Sometimes this situation can go on for years – your anger remains locked inside you and is never expressed.

Physical effects of repressing anger

Not giving outward expression to angry feelings may seem like the way to a harmonious stress-free life, but in fact the opposite is true. Not only is bottled-up anger likely to increase your angry feelings, possibly resulting at some point in an almighty explosion of rage, but the effort of repressing feelings over a long period of time is linked to a number of ailments. You may think that you are benefiting from not expressing your anger verbally, but in fact your feelings are being expressed through your body's reactions. You are likely to suffer one or more of the following ailments:

- headaches
- muscle tension
- stomach complaints
- loss of libido
- eating disorders
- depression of your immune system

- skin disorders
- chest pains.

Mental and psychological effects of mismanaging anger

Not handling anger effectively can affect your well-being and your relationships. It can lead to a cynical outlook on life, in which you are primed to always look for the worst in people or situations. You may become suspicious and wary of others, and your relationships may be soured. Your ability to enjoy life is lessened, and your self-esteem plummets. Feelings of guilt, remorse, frustration, inadequacy and self-blame colour the way you see yourself and others, and act as stumbling-blocks to enjoyable and fulfilling relationships.

If you are constantly ruled by the emotional pressure of anger, expressed or unexpressed, your ability to think clearly and rationally will be undermined, and your potential to be creative and proactive in problem-solving may be diminished. It is hard to focus clearly on issues if you are tense and wound up. You may find that this affects your personal and work life.

Not only feelings, but behaviour is affected by the constant presence of anger. People whose anger is not managed well can behave in edgy and unpredictable ways, causing others to view them warily. This can lead to lack of communication, isolation, withdrawal.

Another danger of unresolved or suppressed anger is that it is linked to anxiety and depression. It can also cause addictive or compulsive behaviour.

Is anger a problem for you?

What if, against your better judgement, you just lose your temper now and again? Perhaps you let rip at home when family members aren't pulling their weight, or sound off at a motorist who steals your parking space. What about the times when you are so frustrated by being put on hold yet again when you want to speak to someone on the phone, or by having taken time off for a delivery which doesn't arrive, that you just can't help flaring up in a temper?

The occasional outbreak isn't going to do any harm – nobody's perfect. In fact, a short controlled expression of anger can do some good, when the burst of adrenalin makes us focused and clear-headed. We all react impulsively and even unfairly now and again. Rather than over-react and beat ourselves up for this kind of behaviour, it is far better to regret these incidents and learn from them without losing our sense of proportion or damaging our self-esteem. What we can do is channel the energy that anger produces into productive channels.

On the other hand, what if, although you feel angry, you just can't express these feelings? Perhaps you bite back the words and pretend that nothing is wrong. Perhaps you feel anger, but call it by another name. There are occasions, of course, when you may choose not to reveal your feelings, but if you constantly stifle and refuse to acknowledge them, your anger is likely to turn inwards and become a real problem for yourself and for others.

Anger is a problem when:

- your anger is very quickly kindled;
- you get angry often;
- you shout at people;
- your anger lasts for a long time;
- you lose control;
- you become aggressive, physically or verbally;
- your anger is linked with violence;
- your anger is linked with alcohol;
- your anger is linked with drugs;
- your anger and frustration are turned on yourself;
- your relationships are damaged;
- your body is always tensed for action;
- you don't feel good about the way you are handling your feelings;
- you don't acknowledge your angry feelings;
- you are scared of expressing feelings of anger;
- you feel angry and powerless;
- you use anger to keep other feelings at bay;
- you hold grudges;
- you focus on getting revenge;
- you want to exert your power over others;
- anger stops you thinking clearly and affects your judgement;
- you feel guilty about your anger;

- your anger is out of all proportion to the event that occasioned it;
- getting angry is the only way you have of dealing with difficult situations;
- you avoid people and situations because you will get angry;
- people avoid you because of your anger.

Short-term gains, long-term losses

Sometimes anger seems to be not just the only choice, but the one which will help us get what we want. A forceful display of aggression can cause the other person to back down; getting your own back on someone by doing or saying something hurtful can feel very satisfying; getting angry can make you feel in charge and in control of the situation. Similarly, keeping quiet about your angry feelings can buy a measure of peace and quiet, and avoid rows and unpleasantness.

These perceived advantages are not real benefits. They may give an immediate sense of satisfaction, but this is short-lived. Mismanaged anger does nothing to solve problems or to improve situations. It causes harm, to ourselves and to others in our lives.

The advantages of healthy and positive anger

There are ways of managing anger which do not depend on violent outbursts or on bottling it up. Anger which is justified and expressed appropriately to the right person or persons in the right way is healthy and positive. Direct, assertive expressions of anger, far from damaging relationships, actually improve them through enhanced communication and honesty.

Justified anger, expressed appropriately, has many benefits:

- It is energizing and vitalizing.
- It alerts us to threat.
- It helps us to protect ourselves.
- It increases self-knowledge and knowledge of others.
- It deepens trust and understanding.
- It helps us to keep in touch with our beliefs and values.

- It helps us to focus on what really matters.
- It can lead to constructive action.

You may notice that none of these benefits relates to our everyday images of angry behaviour. The advantages of recognizing, harnessing and channelling our anger into appropriate behaviour and actions are not gained through displays of aggression or violence. Rather, we can use our anger to help us to develop skills of communication and qualities of persistence, determination, understanding and compassion. We can learn to be forceful without being aggressive, and to be persuasive without being wheedling or bullying. Anger can be the starting point to help us to sharpen our ability to negotiate and to communicate in order to find solutions and ways of living calmly.

What we need to do is to learn how to manage our anger response and make decisions about how to express our feelings, decisions which are based on sound beliefs and clear thinking. To do this we have to acknowledge the strength and the purpose of our automatic responses, but we have to be able to control our reactions so that we are not catapulted into unwary action by the fierce emotions and hormonal energy that invade our bodies and minds.

3

The real causes of anger and how to deal with them

We become angry with other people when they hurt or frustrate us or let us down. Situations wind us up – queues, traffic jams, the car not starting, the computer crashing, the kids squabbling. We get angry when we hear stories about people who cheat or are cruel. We say things like 'It makes my blood boil' and 'It just made me see red', 'it' being the circumstances or the example which has got us going.

Exercise 3.1: What makes you angry?

Think about the things that annoy you or set you off in a rage.

Who and what makes you angry? Try to identify the occasions and situations which spark your anger or annoyance. See if any of the following strike a chord with you. Beside each example, on a scale of 1 to 10, mark the strength of your reaction to the situation, where 1 is mildly annoyed and 10 is very angry.

Being denied something I want	1 2 3 4 5 6 7 8 9 10
Being put down by someone	1 2 3 4 5 6 7 8 9 10
People not pulling their weight	1 2 3 4 5 6 7 8 9 10
Being ignored	1 2 3 4 5 6 7 8 9 10
People breaking promises or letting me down	1 2 3 4 5 6 7 8 9 10
Children arguing and fighting	1 2 3 4 5 6 7 8 9 10
Other motorists	1 2 3 4 5 6 7 8 9 10
Public transport not working	1 2 3 4 5 6 7 8 9 10
Injustice	1 2 3 4 5 6 7 8 9 10
Dishonesty	1 2 3 4 5 6 7 8 9 10
People getting away with things	1 2 3 4 5 6 7 8 9 10
Computers and technology not working	1 2 3 4 5 6 7 8 9 10
Being criticized	1 2 3 4 5 6 7 8 9 10
People trying to control me	1 2 3 4 5 6 7 8 9 10
Noise	1 2 3 4 5 6 7 8 9 10

Being lied to	1 2 3 4 5 6 7 8 9 10
Being taken for granted	1 2 3 4 5 6 7 8 9 10
Being criticized	1 2 3 4 5 6 7 8 9 10
Being kept waiting	1 2 3 4 5 6 7 8 9 10
When my feelings aren't considered	1 2 3 4 5 6 7 8 9 10
Being told what to do	1 2 3 4 5 6 7 8 9 10
Not being listened to	1 2 3 4 5 6 7 8 9 10
Racist or homophobic behaviour	1 2 3 4 5 6 7 8 9 10
Being put on hold on the phone	1 2 3 4 5 6 7 8 9 10
Not being able to get through to the right person	1 2 3 4 5 6 7 8 9 10

Add your own ideas:

_____

_____

_____

It's not the situation, it's us

We talk about anger as if it is caused by something outside ourselves. We think that there is an inevitable chain of events in which one of the above incidents occurs and sparks an angry reaction, and there we are, in the grip of an emotion we didn't have a minute ago, absolutely unable to do anything about it.

In fact, although external events trigger reactions, they are not the cause of our anger. Anger comes from ourselves, from the way that we perceive events and the thoughts that we have about them.

Anger is actually not our first response to a threat or trigger – our first response is a thought. The thought can occur so quickly that we are hardly aware of it, and the thought, or perception, is framed by a number of variables such as our personality, our culture, the particular circumstances. These thoughts which provoke our angry responses may reflect sound and accurate interpretations of the situation. Often, though, our way of thinking about and interpreting events is biased and inaccurate, and our anger is caused by our own way of thinking, our own mindset, which is stuck in a particular mode.

Some of the ways in which our own thoughts make us angry are:

Unrealistic expectations

Much of our anger and frustration comes from expectations which are unlikely to be met. These expectations can be focused on ourselves, on other people and their behaviour, on occasions and events. You may well have a store of ideas and beliefs about how you, other people and the world should be. Your own code of behaviour and your own set of values have evolved throughout your life, formed and influenced by your upbringing, education, your peer group, the significant role models in your life. Consciously or unconsciously, you apply these values to yourself and to others, and set up expectations which are unlikely to be met all of the time. Sometimes the higher the expectations we have, the greater the intensity of our anger when we are disappointed. This is not to say that it's a bad idea to hope for the best and to have high ideals, but that it is a good idea to keep an eye on reality and accept that absolute perfection would be lovely but is usually not attainable. Human beings, including ourselves, aren't perfect, and neither is the world in which we live.

Expectations of ourselves

If we expect too much of ourselves, we end up feeling angry because we have fallen short of the ideals to which we aspire. Sometimes we may not even be aware of the pressure we put ourselves under in order to achieve non-achievable goals.

For many women, the constant attempt to be perfect in every area of our lives – as mothers, as daughters, in our jobs and careers, in our bodies and our appearance, in our social lives – leads to constant failures and disappointments. Our anger with ourselves for these 'failures' can be expressed in numerous ways. Sometimes we blame ourselves for being so useless, as we see it, and for letting ourselves down. Our disappointment in ourselves then damages our self-esteem, causing us to feel even more depressed about our perceived failures and inabilities.

You may have particular areas of your life and your behaviour in which you take pride in maintaining a high ideal. You might demand of yourself that you are never late for an appointment, or that you always tidy the house before you go out, or that you always succeed in everything you do. Of course, there is nothing wrong with having high standards, but if your expectations are unrealistically high you are putting yourself under the kind of pressure which is likely to result in anger and stress.

The pizza problem

Laura is very concerned that her children should have a healthy and nutritious diet.

She has made it a rule for herself that she will never use ready-made meals, but will cook from scratch, using fresh ingredients, so that she knows exactly what they are eating. It's hard to stick to this always, though, and sometimes Laura is just so pressed for time that they have to make do with something like frozen pizza or chicken nuggets. On these occasions, Laura feels that she has failed and let herself down. This makes her angry with herself, and she is out of sorts and niggly all evening.

Exercise 3.2: Do you have unrealistic self-expectations?

Complete these statements with all the examples that occur to you.

1 I think that with my family
   (a) I should

   _____

   (b) I should

   _____

   (c) I should

   _____

   (d) I should

   _____

2 I think that with my spouse or partner
   (a) I should

   _____

   (b) I should

   _____

   (c) I should

   _____

   (d) I should

   _____

3 I think that at work

(a) I should

_____

(b) I should

_____

(c) I should

_____

(d) I should

_____

4 I think that to have an acceptable appearance

(a) I should

_____

(b) I should

_____

(c) I should

_____

(d) I should

_____

5 I think that with my friends and social groups

(a) I should

_____

(b) I should

_____

(c) I should

_____

(d) I should

_____

6 I think that in my behaviour in public

(a) I should

_____

(b) I should

_____

(c) I should

_____

(d) I should

_____

Expectations of others

You might also have unrealistic expectations about how other people should behave. Some of these expectations will stem from the values that are important to you, and may well reflect the demands you make of yourself. In these cases we get angry with people who don't live up to the standards that we, consciously or unconsciously, have imposed on them as well as on ourselves. You might have ideas about how a family 'should' behave towards each other, for example, and this could fuel your anger when members of your family quarrel or act selfishly or refuse to share. If you think that honesty and integrity are qualities that should be displayed in the workplace, you may become angry when you come across cheating or deception.

Your ideas about people's behaviour may make perfect sense and be morally sound – but that isn't the point. What matters is that you are imposing your own ideas on others and are becoming angry when these ideas are not shared or reflected in the actions of others.

Politeness costs nothing

Marnie's anger is readily ignited when she feels that people aren't behaving as they ought to. She believes in courtesy and politeness, and becomes outraged when she encounters surly or grumpy behaviour from members of her family or from people who behave rudely in public. Today someone barged past her in the narrow entrance to the supermarket and didn't even look to see if she was all right, then she had to manoeuvre her way past a couple of people who were standing chatting in the middle of the aisle, blocking everyone's way. Marnie fumes and frets with annoyance. Everyone should be capable of basic courtesy, Marnie thinks, and she is constantly angry and disappointed when this proves to be too much to expect from others.

Exercise 3.3: Do you have unrealistic expectations of other people?

1 I think my family should ...

   (a) _____

   (b) _____

   (c) _____

   (d) _____

2 I think that my spouse or partner should ...

(a) _____

(b) _____

(c) _____

(d) _____

3 I think that people I work with should ...

(a) _____

(b) _____

(c) _____

(d) _____

4 I think that my friends and people in my social groups should ...

(a) _____

(b) _____

(c) _____

(d) _____

5 I think that people in public positions should ...

(a) _____

(b) _____

(c) _____

(d) _____

Think of an occasion or occasions when you became angry at yourself or at others for failing to live up to your expectations.

What happened	*My feelings*
1	
2	
3	

Expectations of events

When we desperately want things to go right, perhaps a holiday or a social occasion, or a meeting or a presentation at work, we can invest so much in our expectations that we almost build in inevitable disappointment. Then our disappointment or frustration can lead to anger and rows.

The perfect wedding celebration

Lucy is planning her wedding. It will be a big event, taking place a year from now. The celebration will begin with the hen party, a weekend in a spa with her bridesmaids and some close friends. On the day itself there will be a church service, followed by a reception at home in a marquee in the garden, with a live band and a disco rounding up the evening. Lucy is determined that this big day will be absolutely perfect in every respect, and lots of money and hours are being invested to create the day that she wants.

Inevitably, throughout the planning period there are a few setbacks and disappointments. Two of her friends say that they can't afford the spa weekend. The photographer Lucy particularly wanted is already booked; she can't find just the right shade of pink for the bridesmaids' dresses; there are arguments about the guest list. Whenever something like this occurs, Lucy gets very angry and upset. She cries with frustration and says that her day is going to be ruined. She hangs on to an image of perfection in which every aspect of the wedding should be exactly as she envisages it, and all she succeeds in doing is fuelling her anger and creating misery for herself and the others involved.

Exercise 3.4: Do you have fixed ideas?

You might have fixed ideas about what you expect from particular events. It could be that you always want Christmas Day to be perfect, or that you want planned occasions like celebrations or events at work to turn out exactly as you intended.

Think of an occasion or occasions when your expectations of an event were not met, and how you reacted.

	Event	Thwarted expectation	My feelings
1			
2			
3			

What we think we're entitled to

Sometimes we become angry and frustrated because we feel that our rights have been violated. On occasion, this is genuinely the case. Often, however, the rights which we feel are under attack aren't rights at all. They are just ideas we have about circumstances and situations that would be desirable, and that have become embedded in our minds as things we are actually entitled to.

Of course, social conventions and legal frameworks do protect some of these aspects of our lives to some extent, but our false ideas about what we have by right can create feelings of anger that we are being done out of something which is rightfully ours.

Exercise 3.5: Assess your feelings of entitlement

To what extent do you instinctively feel that you are entitled to:

	A lot	A little	Not at all
Respect from your family	☐	☐	☐
Respect from others	☐	☐	☐
Consideration of your feelings	☐	☐	☐
A job that you like	☐	☐	☐
Reliable transport	☐	☐	☐
Good service	☐	☐	☐
Be able to buy things you want	☐	☐	☐
Be able to afford things you want	☐	☐	☐
A good doctor/dentist	☐	☐	☐
Courtesy	☐	☐	☐
Privacy	☐	☐	☐
Peace and quiet	☐	☐	☐
Use your mobile phone where and when you choose	☐	☐	☐
Speak your mind	☐	☐	☐
Profit from the housing market	☐	☐	☐
A worry-free existence	☐	☐	☐
Recognition for good work	☐	☐	☐
The kind of holiday you like	☐	☐	☐
Use your free time as you choose	☐	☐	☐

Add your own ideas:

_____

_____

_____

Exercise 3.6: Feeling thwarted

Think of three occasions when you became angry because you were thwarted in something that you felt entitled to.

Occasion	Right that was denied	How I felt

1 _____

2 _____

3 _____

Mind-reading, making assumptions, jumping to conclusions, taking it personally

We often wind ourselves up unnecessarily through making false assumptions about people's behaviour and motives. If a work colleague doesn't say hallo, it's a personal slight; if a friend doesn't respond to your email or phone message, you're not important to him or her; if your mother says you look well, you think she means you've put on weight. We see two people whispering and assume they are talking about us.

You might have noticed how in these situations we rarely give the benefit of the doubt. We take things personally. We assume that there is personal hostility towards us, and that people are deliberately hurting us. We blame others or ourselves for the anger that this creates.

> ### She did that on purpose
> Jenny and Vicki audition for the same role in their amateur dramatic society, and Jenny gets the part. On the first night of the performance Vicki treads on the hem of Jenny's dress and tears it quite badly. 'She did that on purpose to rattle me,' thinks Jenny. 'She resents me for having this part, and she wants to see me make a mess of it.'
>
> Jenny assumes that she knows what is going on in Vicki's mind, and that Vicki's action was deliberate. She simmers with anger every time she thinks about it.

Exercise 3.7: Wrong assumptions

Think of three occasions on which you made wrong assumptions about someone's behaviour.

	Occasion	*What I assumed*
1		
2		
3		

Making everything a catastrophe

Minor annoyances and irritations can become huge causes of anger if our way of thinking about them and describing them makes them worse than they are. We can wind ourselves up by exaggerating how awful something is. Of course, now and again we want to make a bit of a story describing a holiday which turned into a disaster because we were let down by the travel company, or outlining the unbelievable incompetence of some of our work colleagues, or illustrating the incredible insensitivity of our outspoken mother-in-law. The danger is that the exaggeration becomes the truth, and the situation changes in the telling, so that we can end up even more angry and outraged than we were in the first place. The language we use and our style of retelling or thinking about the situation can increase our feelings of anger out of all proportion to the situation that gave rise to them. We turn everything into a disaster or a catastrophe, and our angry emotions run high even when the event is over.

This is the end

Suzi has ordered the wrong flowers for the function on Wednesday. 'This is absolutely awful,' she thinks. 'How can I have been so incredibly stupid? I'll never get another assignment. My name will be mud.'

Exercise 3.8: Disasters and catastrophes

Think of three events which you have mentally or verbally classified as disastrous or catastrophic.

What happened	How I described it
1	
2	
3	

Seeing only the negative

If you only see the negative aspects of a situation and are unable to have a balanced view, you end up being always ready to attack or be attacked. You discount anything good and focus instead on what you perceive as wrong and undesirable, and you can allow one negative point, one disappointment, to dominate your judgement of the whole thing.

That spoils everything

Wendy and Mick have had an enjoyable day with friends at the coast. On the way home they are stuck in a traffic jam for half an hour. 'Just when everything had gone so well,' says Wendy. 'The day is spoilt now.' She is tetchy for the rest of the evening.

The next day they have asked an estate agent for a valuation on their flat. He makes approving comments about the accommodation and its saleability, and says that the kitchen would be described as in need of updating.

'That's it!' Wendy explodes. 'You heard him – we'll never sell this place with the kitchen the way it is.'

Exercise 3.9: Negative thinking

Think of three occasions which you think of in totally negative terms.

	Occasion	What was wrong/I didn't like
1		
2		
3		

Making choices about dealing with anger

These ways of thinking about people and events have probably become automatic, so that you may hardly recognize their connection to your anger. Often we do not realize that anger is not something caused by external events, but is primarily linked to the way that we think. You also may not recognize that some of your thoughts are not realistic, and that they indicate a skewed version of situations. They are habits of thinking which underpin our view of the world and are so much a part of us that we don't stop to challenge them. Yet these distorted thoughts give rise to feelings of anger, frustration and resentment, and are at the root of mismanaged anger.

Taking responsibility for managing your angry moods and

responses will greatly enhance your confidence and self-esteem. To acknowledge that we can take charge of our thoughts and influence our emotions is extraordinarily invigorating and is the path to a calmer, more stress-free life. Not rushing to blame others for the way we feel means that we take away their power to hurt us. Eleanor Roosevelt said that no one can be made to feel inferior without their consent. In other words, no one can make you feel or react in a certain way. Of course, others provide the stimulus and others provoke a reaction – but you can make sure that your reaction isn't an automatic response to a situation. No one can 'make' you cry – you cry as a result of what has been done or said. No one can 'make' you feel mad – you feel mad as a result of your thoughts about a situation. The only person who can 'make' you angry is yourself – and this is what we do, over and over again.

Getting rid of thoughts that fuel our anger

Anger is not something over which we have no control: anger is a choice. This seems to be far from the case when we experience that overwhelming surge of adrenalin which invades our body and makes us want to hit out at whatever is threatening or causing us pain, but we can manage and control our response by choosing how to think about the event and how to respond to what is triggering our anger. This approach to managing our emotions is based on cognitive behavioural therapy. The basis of this therapy is that our anger is triggered by a situation which gives rise to automatic thoughts about the dangers and consequences of the situation. These thoughts then arouse anger and hostility. What we can do is stop this sequence of events by altering our perspective and changing the way that we think about people and situations. We can challenge these unhelpful habits of thought and replace them with more calming responses. Doing this helps us to break the connection between the trigger, the thought and the eruption of anger, and is one of the key elements in learning to manage anger.

Thinking more realistically

Laura would be calmer if she thought: 'Ideally I would like to give my kids only home-made food. Practically, that isn't always possible. Overall, they have a good diet.'

Lucy would enjoy her wedding preparations much more if she kept on an even keel by thinking: 'I'm doing everything possible to create the perfect day, and there are some things over which I have no control. I can accept that perhaps some things won't turn out exactly as planned, but there is no point in getting angry and allowing frustration to spoil the enjoyment of a happy occasion.'

Marnie would be less grumpy and irritable if she thought: 'I think politeness is important. It would be good if everyone felt the same way as I do, but other people are entitled to behave in a different way. I will continue to be courteous, no matter how others behave.'

If you recognize that you expect too much of yourself, of other people and of events, you are liable to become frustrated and angry when your expectations aren't met. Try to alter your way of thinking so that you lessen the pressure on yourself. This doesn't mean that you should change your whole way of looking at the world, but just that you may benefit from changing some of the habits of thought which may be fuelling your anger.

Instead of thinking: 'I've got to be the perfect mother', think: 'I will be the best mother that I can be. I won't get everything right all the time.'

Instead of thinking: 'It's not fair that I work so hard and don't earn as much as other people', think: 'The world isn't fair, and I have to expect inequality. I could look for ways of earning more money, but I might as well accept that there will be always those who make more than I do. There is no point in being angry about that.'

Exercise 3.10: Unrealistic expectations

Choose three of your thoughts which are based on unrealistic expectations. Change them to more helpful ways of thinking.

	Unrealistic thought	*Realistic thought*
1		
2		
3		

How to ease up on unrealistic expectations

- Accept that no one is perfect.
- Accept that you have no right to impose your standards on others.
- Stop saying 'should' and 'must'.
- Use expressions such as 'I'd like' or 'I'd prefer'.
- Enjoy looking forward to events.
- Be optimistic about outcomes.
- Accept that nothing is guaranteed to be perfect.
- Resolve to enjoy the occasion even if it doesn't go entirely to plan.

How to stop making assumptions and avoid the mind-reading trap

Jenny would not be angry if she thought: 'Vicki probably stood on my dress by accident. After all, she hasn't actually done or said anything to make me think that she resents my getting the part.'

If you often assume that you know what people are thinking or you know what their motives are, you could try altering your perspective to accommodate other explanations for people's behaviour.

Instead of thinking: 'Mona is frowning. She must have read my report', think: 'Mona could be frowning for a number of reasons. I won't know what she thinks of my report until we discuss it.'

Instead of thinking: 'Kit left his breakfast things on the table deliberately to annoy me', think: 'He may have been in a hurry, or he may have just forgotten to clear up. I'll talk to him about it.'

Instead of thinking: 'I could tell she didn't really like my new hair colour', think: 'I'm not quite sure exactly what she thought. If I want to know, I'll ask her.'

Ask yourself, 'Could I be wrong?' Remind yourself that there may be several reasons for people's behaviour

Practise by observing people at home or at work when they act in ways which you think of as showing hostility. You might think that someone is giving you a dirty look, or that they are ignoring you, or that they did something to harm you on purpose. Come up with at least three possible explanations for their behaviour. It could be that the person:

- was feeling distracted and miles away;
- made a genuine mistake;
- had a pounding headache;
- had a hangover.

Add your own ideas:

_____

_____

_____

Exercise 3.11: Your assumptions

Choose three assumptions that you made recently. Write down the thought you had, and replace it with a possible alternative.

	How someone behaved	My assumption	Alternative explanation
1			
2			
3			

How to stop turning everything into a catastrophe

If you tend to exaggerate and make things much worse than they are, get into the habit of seeing blips and stumbling-blocks instead of out-and-out disasters. After all, you didn't really 'nearly die' when you were overheard talking about your boss. It might have been an awkward and embarrassing situation, but it wasn't a near-death experience.

Instead of thinking: 'This is the worst day of my life', think: 'This has been a really difficult day.'

Instead of thinking: 'I'll never get over this', think: 'This is very tough at the moment.'

Instead of thinking: 'I look an absolute mess', think: 'I'm not looking my best at the moment.'

Exercise 3.12: Describing your anger

Choose three occasions when you were angry with somebody or a situation. What words did you use to describe your anger? Choose expressions from the following suggestions to express your anger on that occasion.

the most awful thing   really hate it when
pretty annoying   drives me mad
irritating   don't like it when
a bit frustrating   it's awful
infuriating   can't stand it
disastrous   niggling
incredibly annoying   could have died
wanted to kill him   absolute catastrophe

Add your own ideas:

	Situation	How I described it	How I could describe it
1			
2			
3			

How to keep things in perspective

- Moderate your vocabulary – choose milder expressions when appropriate.
- Ask yourself: 'How much will this matter in a week or a year?'
- Use positive self-talk: 'This is not good, but I'll get over it'; 'This is a mistake. They happen.'

Stopping the negativity

Seeing only the negative is a habit of thought which you can change.

Instead of thinking: 'That mistake ruined the whole effect of the display', think: 'Most things were effective.'

Instead of thinking: 'The evening will be ruined if Martha's late', think: 'I hope Martha will be on time. If she isn't, it will be annoying, but we'll cope.'

Exercise 3.13: Thinking positive

Think of three occasions which you think of in totally negative terms. Identify one or two things that were positive about the occasion.

	Occasion	What was wrong/I didn't like	What was right
1			
2			
3			

The power of reframing

This is a highly effective way of not only controlling your anger but finding something positive in a tense situation. What you do is see the situation from a different point of view and find something good in it instead of focusing on what is bad. Not only does this reduce feelings of anger and hostility, it offers you scope for finding something enjoyable or affirming in what seems to be a grim situation.

Severe delays on the motorway

Danielle and Nathan are driving to their holiday destination in the Lake District on a hot day in August, where they are due to meet up with another family for their first meal of the holiday. They are making good time until the traffic starts to slow and the radio informs them that a queue of several miles is building up and severe delays are expected.

Their thoughts at this point could focus on the frustration and nuisance caused by the delay: they could find their tempers rising, and talk about what an awful start to the holiday, why the highway authorities can't sort these things out more quickly, and how the others will have their evening spoilt if they don't make it in time. Instead, they decide to text their friends to let them know they might be late, and pull off at the next exit and take an hour or two to explore one of the local towns or villages. They will find somewhere more appealing than motorway services for something to eat and drink, and will view the stop as an opportunity to visit somewhere they would otherwise never have seen.

The in-laws' visit

Andrea finds her in-laws' visits very trying. What really gets to her is the way that Dave's mother constantly finds subtle ways of criticizing the way Andrea deals with the children. Andrea decides that she will think about positive, assertive ways of addressing this problem, and will see their next visit as an opportunity to put her communication skills to good effect and build a more open and equal relationship with her mother-in-law.

Exercise 3.14: Reframing in a positive way

Think of three situations which you could reframe in a positive way.

Situation:
Thoughts about it that make me angry:
Reframed thoughts:

Situation:
Thoughts about it that make me angry:
Reframed thoughts:

Situation:
Thoughts about it that make me angry:
Reframed thoughts:

4

Different ways of showing anger

We have looked at the ways in which our anger is triggered, and how patterns of thinking that we all share can influence our angry feelings. But just as we are all subject to different types of distorted thinking, so there is a huge variety in the ways that we experience and express our emotional responses. You may have experienced occasions when you get really annoyed about something and another person just shrugs it off, or times when you find something funny and another person is angry because he or she finds the same thing offensive. You might feel mildly irritated and mutter a few words of complaint when there is a long queue at a ticket office, while your friend might explode with rage and frustration. The way that we respond depends on our individual make-up – our thinking patterns, our patterns of behaviour, the way we were brought up, our childhood experiences, the environment we inhabit, our level of self-management skills. Recognizing how you express anger and assessing the effects of your usual behaviour is a crucial part of learning how to manage anger effectively.

The angry explosion

Explosions occur when something triggers our rage and we are so incensed that we find ourselves lashing out at someone, often hardly aware of our words and actions. Our body is responding in the way that it is primed to deal with a threat. Adrenalin rushes through our bloodstream, our heart thumps, our mouth goes dry and our muscles tense. It is quite likely that, without realizing it, our hands form fists. Angry words fly out, often accompanied by aggressive actions, maybe pointing and jabbing, or punching the air.

Sammi and the credit card statement

Sammi happens to see her partner Graham's credit card statement. She can hardly believe her eyes – they are on an economy drive and have agreed that they will cut down on the amount of money they spend on eating and drinking out. Yet here is the evidence that Graham has run up a hefty bar tab on several occasions in the past month, while she has made all kinds of cutbacks, even doing without her favourite skinny lattes on the way to work. Sammi's anger reaches boiling point very quickly, and she turns on Graham as soon as he comes in. 'I can't believe you!' she explodes. 'How could you be so selfish!' She rants at Graham for a good few minutes, telling him that he can't be trusted and that he only thinks of himself, and that there's no point in them agreeing about anything because he will just go behind her back and do what he likes ... Her voice gets higher and higher. She is shaking with rage, and she ends up in tears.

The short-term effects of letting off steam can be satisfying. The immediate release of tension and the physical high we experience when we express our feelings forcefully are heady and invigorating, and we may feel that we have almost literally 'got something off our chest'. However, in the long term, this kind of outburst has more costs than benefits. When we run with our angry feelings and let rip with words and actions, we are behaving without judgement and without control. We are allowing our emotions to smother our ability to think and behave rationally, and although the effect on the immediate situation may be satisfying, we have not dealt with the problem, and it is very likely that we have damaged a relationship and lost both self-respect and the respect of others. Expressing our anger in a more measured and controlled way may seem low-key and lacking drama, but it is the route to the ultimate satisfaction of improved relationships, strong self-respect and being responsible for our own emotional and physical well-being.

Are you an exploder?

Do you express your angry feelings by:

- speaking or shouting very loudly?
- being physically aggressive?
- becoming very angry very quickly?
- not caring or being aware of what you say?

- unleashing the power of your feelings on to the other person?
- doing and saying things in the heat of the moment which you later regret?

Add your own examples:

_____

_____

_____

Exercise 4.1: Expressing anger

Think of a few times when you experienced an explosion of anger. Jot down the kind of words that you used, what your actions were, and a brief description of your feelings at the time. What was the result of your outburst?

	Situation	What I said	What I did	How I felt	Outcome
1					
2					
3					

Better ways of dealing with explosive moments

When you feel on the brink of a furious outburst, rather than build yourself up to an explosion, try these ideas:

- Take time to think before you speak.
- Do some breathing and relaxation exercises to help you to stay calm.
- Walk away from the situation or from the person if you need to.
- Do something physical to work off your hostility.
- Figure out exactly what is the source of your anger.
- Decide if it is something you need to address.
- Work out what you want to say.
- Choose a time and a place which will help you to express your anger forcefully and appropriately.

Managing your feelings in these ways will help you to keep control of your emotions and of your words. Anger is too valuable to be wasted in an outburst which in the end achieves nothing and may in fact have the opposite effect of what you intend. The fierceness of your emotions tells you that something is wrong, so use this message to help you identify and communicate what you want to change.

Venting your anger

You may have experienced occasions when you feel so wound up about a situation that you just need the emotional release of screaming or shouting or hitting something. You feel the urge to let off steam safely, without directing your anger at individuals.

Amina lets it all out
Amina is infuriated with her supervisor at work, who has refused to let her have time off for a personal appointment. There have been a few similar encounters with this manager. Amina bottles up her anger until she gets home, then she stomps around the sitting room, shouting and swearing, and punches the cushions on the sofa until she feels exhausted. Later on she tells her partner about the incident and about how she dealt with her feelings.

'Do you feel better now?' he asks.

Amina starts to say yes, she does, then she stops and says, 'I just feel tired. And I'm still angry.'

The trouble with venting anger in this way is that it does nothing to address the situation which has caused it, and it actually helps to fuel your feelings rather than calm them. Strategies such as sounding off to a friend, hitting a cushion or finding a place where you can shout and scream may seem like safe and effective ways of handling your angry feelings, but all you are doing is focusing on the very emotion which is making you feel bad.

Women are sometimes encouraged to express their anger like this, as an antidote to years of cultural conditioning which has resulted in their anger being bottled up, and it can feel powerful and therapeutic to acknowledge and give vent to rage. In the long run, though, it is much healthier to address the situation and identify the source of your anger so that you can decide how to deal with it. Venting may be a satisfying release of emotion, but it is not good anger management.

Are you a 'venter'?

Do you express your angry feelings by:

- shouting, swearing, hitting out in a 'safe' context?
- throwing something?
- letting it all out to a sympathetic friend over a glass of wine?
- giving physical expression to your anger in a 'safe' context?
- giving verbal expression to your anger in a 'safe' context?

Add your own examples:

_____

_____

_____

Exercise 4.2: How did you vent your anger?

Think of a few times when you vented your anger in this way. Jot down the kind of words that you used, what your actions were, and a brief description of your feelings at the time. What was the result of your 'venting' experience?

	Situation	What I said	What I did	How I felt	Outcome
1					
2					
3					

Better ways of venting your anger

When you feel that you are bursting with anger and frustration and need a short sharp release for your emotional tension, you could try:

- going for a jog or a run;
- going for a power walk;
- putting on some upbeat music that you like and dancing round the room;
- doing some serious cleaning – scrubbing a floor, cleaning all the windows;
- doing some active gardening.

Add your own examples:

_____

_____

_____

Channelling your emotional energy into this kind of physical activity is a positive way of managing anger. It will release your muscle tension and produce hormones which have a feel-good effect. Be careful, though – this strategy will be counter-productive if you accompany your activity with going over and over what happened, or dwelling on angry thoughts. Instead, pick some calming thoughts and phrases and repeat them over and over again to the rhythm of your movements.

Repressing your anger

Many women bottle up their anger. Repressing your feelings in this way is different from suppressing anger, or keeping it in until you can express it positively and safely. By repressing we mean burying your feelings, sometimes to such an extent that you deny that you have them. It may be that we prefer to think that we don't have these angry feelings, and so deny what is happening, or give another name to our emotional turmoil. We may not even realize that the emotion we are experiencing is anger.

We repress anger for a number of reasons. Sometimes we do it because we are afraid of our angry feelings, and of the emotions that will be revealed if we talk about what is inside us. We may be scared of the strength of our emotions; we may be scared of what revealing our anger may lead to. We may feel too intimidated to speak out. We may think that anger means confrontation, and that is something that we can't handle.

Do you bottle up your anger?

You might find it comparatively easy to be angry with certain people in your life, but there may be other contexts in which you find it very difficult or impossible to talk about the way that you feel.

Exercise 4.3: How hard is it to express your anger?

How difficult do you find it to express your anger:

	Very hard	Quite hard	Not a problem
To your husband or partner	☐	☐	☐
To your children	☐	☐	☐
In front of your children	☐	☐	☐
To a friend	☐	☐	☐
To your parents	☐	☐	☐
To a work colleague	☐	☐	☐
To your boss at work	☐	☐	☐
To someone who has given you poor service	☐	☐	☐
To someone who has been rude to you	☐	☐	☐
To someone who has hurt you	☐	☐	☐

Add your own examples:

_____

_____

_____

If you can't express your anger but let it seethe away inside you, it is more than likely to emerge anyway in a disguised form. Repressed anger is often revealed in behaviour that isn't overtly hostile, but which may mask deep-rooted feelings of resentment and rage. There are different ways in which we give indirect expression to our anger. Often this is not done consciously, and we may be unaware of the strategies we employ to cover up our real feelings.

Some strategies we use to cover up angry feelings

Pretending it's no big deal

Melissa's late again

Sian likes her evening out with Melissa. Melissa is bubbly and full of life, and has a way of lifting Sian's spirits at the end of a hard day. The problem is that Melissa is never on time. Sian makes a real effort to keep to the time agreed, but more often than not, just as she's arriving, she gets a text saying that Melissa will be late. This really annoys Sian, and she tries to let Melissa know this with little comments:

'It would be nice if you could let me know in advance if you're running late, but not to worry.'
'Oh well, better late than never.'
'At least you're here now.'
'I was beginning to think my watch was wrong.'

Sian feels that it would be hurtful and unfriendly to tell Melissa that she is annoyed and feels taken for granted by her unpunctuality, and her feelings of resentment grow and threaten to spoil the friendship.

Being sarcastic

Grounding Jasmine

Joanne has grounded Jasmine for a week because she came in very late and didn't text home to say where she was. Jasmine told her father that she thought Joanne was being unfair. He backed their daughter up and said that she wasn't grounded any more. Joanne is furious. She says things like:

'Oh, I must have imagined that I had grounded her.'
'Silly me, to think that you would support me.'

These indirect statements of anger do not address the issue and they mean that Joanne's real feelings are not heeded. She makes it easy for her point of view to be ignored, and this increases her internal anger.

Getting your own back

Kirsten's revenge

Kirsten is angry with her work colleague Danny. He forgot to pass on a message and so she was late for an important meeting. Recently there have been several similar occasions when he has not passed on information, and she's had enough of it. Kirsten broods about Danny's behaviour, and sees her chance to get back at him when he leaves his phone on his desk when he goes to speak to someone for a few minutes. Kirsten slips his phone into a drawer and piles papers on top of it. She enjoys watching Danny's panic and frustration as he frantically searches for the phone. 'Serves him right,' she thinks.

Kirsten's behaviour actually fuels her anger. She chooses not to speak to Danny about these incidents, and instead works herself up into an angry state, thinking that he is behaving on purpose to cause trouble for her. The satisfaction of creating a bit of trouble for him is short-lived and rather than addressing the problem makes things worse by cementing hostility.

The silent treatment

Mavis turns a cold shoulder

Mavis is angry with Barry because he promised to mow the lawn at the weekend, and now it's Sunday evening and the job hasn't been done. She doesn't tell him what is annoying her, but just freezes him out. She doesn't respond to anything he says, and only shrugs when he asks her what's wrong. Mavis thinks that Barry ought to realize what's bugging her, and she isn't going to make it easy by telling him how she is feeling. As the evening goes on she gets more and more angry, but she cannot bring herself to communicate this directly.

Mavis deliberately creates an atmosphere of uncertainty and tension to let Barry know that she is angry. Her way of dealing with the situation suggests that she doesn't want to stop being annoyed about the uncut lawn, but just wants to make things difficult for Barry. She wants him to feel guilty.

Do you mask your anger?

Do you:

- make a joke or laugh it off when a comment or action has hurt you?
- pretend not to be annoyed about something that really gets to you?
- make sarcastic comments about behaviour that annoys you?
- smile when you're feeling angry?
- find excuses for other people's hurtful behaviour?
- bring up the little things that are on your mind but don't approach the big issues?
- minimize the hurt that you feel?
- go over and over in your head conversations that have upset you?
- find a way of getting back at someone you are angry with?
- go over things that you wish you had said or done?
- engage in sabotaging behaviour – keeping back information, being deliberately late, misunderstanding on purpose?
- turn on the tears?
- try to make others feel guilty?

Add your own ideas:

_____

_____

_____

Exercise 4.4: Indirect signs of anger

Think of a few times when you were angry and showed it in an indirect way. Jot down the kind of words that you used, what your actions were, and a brief description of your feelings at the time. What was the result of your actions?

	Situation	What I said	What I did	How I felt	Outcome
1					
2					
3					

Better ways of handling bottled-up anger

- Decide what it is that you are angry about.
- Say the words, 'I am angry because ...'
- Decide if you need to say these words to someone.
- Learn how to communicate your anger assertively.

5

Using anger to your advantage

Your anger tells you something. It is a signal that something is wrong in your world, that you are feeling hurt in some way. Try to regard your angry reactions as part of an alert system, drawing your attention to things that you need to deal with in order to live peacefully. Use your emotional response to guide you to think about ways in which you can make the situation more bearable. If channelled in this way, anger is not something to be feared but a useful part of your emotional make-up, something to be welcomed as a warning sign.

Anger and self-knowledge

How anger helps you to understand yourself

Anger can be a starting point for increasing your self-awareness and self-knowledge. Working out why you are angry with certain people and why you get worked up in certain situations shines a light on your relationships, on your attitudes, on your motivation, on what really matters to you. Recognizing the source of your hostility and any patterns in your angry reactions will help you to manage your feelings effectively. Your relationships and interactions with others will benefit from your enhanced awareness, as they will not be soured by misplaced and misdirected anger.

What are you really angry about?

The anger response is so quick and so automatic that we can direct our annoyance at the person or the situation which is its immediate trigger without stopping to examine the real source of our feelings. In fact, the emotions that have been aroused may be connected to someone or something else entirely, perhaps even something from your past. It is very easy to feel angry with the wrong person for the wrong reason, and to miss the real cause of our discomfort. It can be easier to go with the flow of our anger than to stop and identify its real nature, but the process of unravelling and identifying the true nature of our emotional reaction, though it may be painful, can be valuable and helpful in terms of our personal growth and awareness.

The parent–teacher meeting

Judy has experienced a very uncomfortable time at her son's parent–teacher consultation evening. Luke has assured her that all his coursework is up to date, but now she knows that he has missed deadlines in several of his subjects. She can feel her anger rising as she hears the same story from teacher after teacher, and she storms home to give Luke a piece of her mind and tell him that he is grounded until he makes up the work. She means to speak calmly and firmly, but she ends up shouting at him, and he goes into his room and slams the door.

Later that evening, still wound up about it, she tells her mother what has happened. 'Why were you so angry with Luke?' her mother asks. 'You know he does his best, but he finds it difficult to keep up. This is nothing new.'

'I know it isn't,' says Judy.

When she calms down, she goes over the evening in her head, and thinks about how she felt at each stage. She realizes that she was so angry not because Luke was behind in his work, but because she felt that she looked stupid in front of his teachers for not knowing that this was the case. Judy's self-esteem has taken a dent, and this is not actually Luke's fault. Her anger at Luke softens into concern, and some legitimate annoyance that he had not told her the real situation.

Judy spends some time thinking about the way she hates feeling that she looks stupid. She realizes how often she fires into an angry response when she is actually feeling put down or diminished in some way. Her anger masks her lack of confidence. Now she can work on building her self-esteem, if she wishes to, and she is able more easily to manage the way that she responds in these situations.

What are you feeling other than anger?

In some ways anger is the easy emotion. It can make us feel self-righteous and justified, and its force can sweep us along so that we lose the ability to think clearly about the cause and nature of our reaction. But anger may be a vehicle for other emotions which could remain unacknowledged. It can mask feelings of guilt, hurt, envy, fear, self-doubt. When you are aware of this happening, once you have identified the feeling that is fuelling your anger, you can work on making that feeling a motivating force for change, or you can manage the feeling so that it does not continue to damage you. For example, if you find that you are making snipey comments about someone's success – say, their financial good fortune or their promotion at work or their clever well-behaved children – you might realize that your attitude is shaped by envy. Once you accept that you are feeling envious, not angry, you can make some choices. You could take some steps to achieve the elements of success over which you have some control, such as applying for promotion yourself instead of just winding yourself up thinking how little the other person deserves such treatment and how unfair the workplace is. If you are envious of things which are outside your grasp, or which you genuinely don't want anyway, you could work on eliminating the irrational thinking which governs your attitude.

Exercise 5.1: Feelings behind my anger

What I felt angry about   What feelings were behind my anger

1 _____

2 _____

3 _____

Are you choosing to stay angry?

Sometimes we choose to remain angry. Although anger is uncomfortable, if it is a familiar emotional state we may be reluctant to let it go. It can give us a hook on which to hang our frustrations and dissatisfactions, and it may feel safer to continue being angry than to face the consequences of change. Sometimes subconsciously we feel that being angry is somehow easier to handle than trying other tactics, such as looking for ways to solve a problem, or making the adjustments to our way of thinking that could enable us to live with whatever it is that is getting to us.

Debbie hangs on to her anger

Debbie's children spend every other weekend with their father and his new partner. When they come home they are full of stories about what a good time they've had. Their father spends a lot of money taking them to theme parks and cinemas, and more often than not they arrive back laden with presents. This makes Debbie very angry – she has no spare money for luxuries, and she resents the fact that the time the children spend with their father is associated with having fun and getting things bought for them. She spends every weekend that the children are away thinking about what they will be doing and how he will be spoiling them, and she works herself up into a state of anger and resentment.

Debbie could try to discuss her feelings with the children's father and express her concerns. She knows it is likely that he spoils the children because he feels guilty about having left them. But Debbie doesn't want to be rational, and she doesn't want to show any understanding. She prefers to feel angry and to nurse her feelings of betrayal and resentment. If she releases these feelings, Debbie thinks, it will be as if she is accepting and condoning his behaviour. So she lets the situation eat away at her, instead of using her anger as a vehicle for positive communication.

What outcome do you want?

If you don't want to continue feeling angry, what emotion do you want to take its place? Sometimes we hang on to anger because, like Debbie, we feel that to relinquish it is as if we are giving in and accepting a situation which we don't like. We may see anger as a matter of principle.

Step outside your anger for a moment, and think about what you want to achieve. You might want:

- to feel that you are in the right;
- to feel happy or happier;
- to feel that you have won;
- to feel calm;
- to feel self-respect;
- to feel in control of yourself;
- to feel in control of someone else;
- to feel aggrieved.

Add your own ideas:

_____

_____

_____

Exercise 5.2: Situations that make you angry

Choose three situations that make you angry. Imagine what would happen if you stopped feeling angry about them. What would happen? What would you feel like?

Situation	My feelings	How I would like to feel
1		
2		
3		

Channelling your anger constructively

Anger as a vehicle for change

Anger can lead to constructive action. It can be the motivating force to propel us into doing something about a situation which disturbs us. This may be on a personal level, when the angry emotions we feel in a relationship, for example, can move us to instigate changes that need to be made. Anger can be the starting point for making improvements in relationships and in furthering and deepening our understanding of our own needs and those of the other people in our lives. On a public or political level, our anger at institutions or governments, at injustice or unfairness, can motivate us to protest or campaign for change. Whatever the situation, we need to harness the energy of our anger and channel it into positive strategies and communication.

How anger can help you to make things happen

In your personal life

When anger tells you that something is wrong in an area of your personal life, it can be the spur to make you do something about it. Niggles and dissatisfactions are part of many relationships, maybe particularly so with those close to us – it's just a part of day-to-day living. However, if you recognize that you are feeling genuine, justified anger, take this feeling seriously. You need to identify the true source of your anger and make some decisions about how to deal with it. It might be a case of managing your own feelings about the person or situation and learning to live with it, or you might need to discuss the issue. Work out what you want to change, what you want to be different, then plan the way that you will raise the issue. Think as well about what you will do if the change does not take place, and your anger continues.

At work

If you find yourself getting angry about a situation at work, take the time to think calmly and analyse just what it is that is getting to you. Perhaps you are being treated unfairly. Maybe you are being overworked, or taken advantage of, or exploited in some way. It could be that a colleague is irritating you and getting under your skin. Think about what your feelings are telling you. Your anger might be caused by frustration and feeling under-valued – is this the spur you need to make you seek promotion or another job? If you get worked up because of poor practices and systems, should you find a way of improving these things? Perhaps you need to look for a position where you are responsible for putting good practice into place. Once you identify the nature of your feelings, you are in a good position to decide what to do.

Exercise 5.3: Taking action

Situation
How I feel about it
How I would like it to be different
What I will do

Situation
How I feel about it
How I would like it to be different
What I will do

Situation
How I feel about it
How I would like it to be different
What I will do

In the public domain

You may find that you get very heated about aspects of daily life which you find irritating and annoying. Sometimes such triggers seem small when you talk about them afterwards, but they can cause the kind of bad mood and general disgruntlement which means that your anger is more easily fired by other events.

Turn it off

Lorraine strongly dislikes piped music in shops and public places. She becomes irritated every time she encounters it, and makes a point of seeking out places which don't have a policy of using background music. This isn't always possible, though. Rather than just moaning about the situation and allowing it to get to her, Lorraine finds out about the groups and organizations which campaign to stop the use of piped music, and signs up as a member. She discovers ways of protesting against its use, and identifies the appropriate people to contact. Using this outlet for her annoyance, and feeling that she is taking a stand on an issue of personal and public concern, enables Lorraine to control her reactions when she encounters this irritant.

Take positive action

You might be constantly angry about local issues such as the state of the roads, or planning permissions, or the closure of certain facilities. There might be some national issues about which you get very worked up, or there may be global concerns that really get to you. If your anger is expressed in the occasional rant or outburst, you might be happy just to make sure that you manage your feelings so that they don't lead to damage to yourself or anyone else. If your anger is deep and intrusive, think about using your energy in a positive way.

Some things you might try:

- Write to your local newspaper.
- Write to a national newspaper.
- Join an organization such as a campaign or pressure group or political party, or a group such as a residents' association, which focuses on the issues which concern you.
- Take part in a radio phone-in, local or national.
- Find internet sites where these issues are discussed.
- Start a campaign group.

Add your own ideas:

_____

_____

_____

Keep a sense of perspective

The purpose of the above activities is to find a positive channel for your anger, not to find ways of fanning its flames. If you don't choose to make fighting for an issue your life's work, make sure that it does not occupy your whole life or become your main interest.

6

Communication skills for tense situations

Many arguments and rows begin and become worse because we don't communicate clearly and positively with each other. Lack of communication skills can cause us to feel angry and frustrated. We know what we want but we can't find ways to say it, and we end up feeling that no one listens to or cares about what we want, and that our needs are never met or even considered. Sometimes we bottle up feelings because we just don't know how to express them, or we are scared that we will come across in a way that we hadn't intended, or that we will say things we will later regret.

Three types of skill are particularly helpful when it comes to communicating in situations which involve anger and hostility:

- the ability to communicate assertively;
- the ability to empathize with other people;
- the ability to listen.

Expressing your anger assertively

You can say how angry you are in a positive and productive way. This doesn't mean that you need to hide or mask your feelings, or turn your anger into something less than it is in order to make it more acceptable or easier for the other person to handle. Nor does it mean that you have to be aggressive in order to get your point across and be taken seriously. An assertive expression of anger consists of the right words, spoken in the right way, to the right person or people, at the right time.

Getting the right words

The most important word here is 'I'. You need to acknowledge and own your feelings, and show that you are taking responsibility for the way you feel. Be clear and direct. Don't say that you're disappointed, or that you feel let down, or claim any other emotion if what you feel is anger. If it is what you feel, say:

'I'm angry.'
'I'm annoyed.'
'I'm absolutely furious.'
'I'm beginning to feel really angry about this.'

Choose words which indicate the nature and extent of your anger. Don't underplay the strength of your feelings, and don't exaggerate them either.

Make the cause of your anger clear

Be as precise as you can about the specific situation which is getting to you:

'I'm angry because you ignored what I had said and went ahead and booked the holiday anyway.'
'This is the third time I have phoned to speak to someone about the situation, and I'm getting really annoyed.'
'What I told you about Katie was said in confidence, as I made clear. Now I find that you have repeated it to several people. You know, Lynn, I'm really angry about that.'

Continuing the conversation

How you continue depends on the outcome that you want. If you just want to let someone know that you are angry or were angry and leave it at that, then don't say too much. Finish with something like:

'I need you to know how I feel.'
'I wanted to make my feelings clear.'
'I'm glad I've let you know how I feel about this.'

Once you have said that, walk away, turn away, do whatever is appropriate to show that it is over. Sometimes it's good to physically separate yourself from the other person so that you get a break from each other. This also prevents the anger you have expressed from seeping into ensuing conversation.

If the issue is something that should be discussed further, you need to use words which show that you are willing to listen to another point of view. An assertive expression of anger shows awareness of the other person and focuses on moving beyond anger to improve the situation or the relationship. Phrases you could use include:

'I know you might see this differently.'
'I understand that you ...'
'I realize that you ...'
'How can we make this better?'
'How can we sort this out?'

If you want to instigate some action, make a clear statement of the outcome you are looking for:

'What I'm asking for is ...'
'What I would like is ...'
'From my point of view, the way forward is ...'

Not being deflected

When you have a particular point that you want to make, or something specific that you want to discuss, be careful not to let the conversation lurch into other areas. When people feel that they are being criticized or that they are under attack they often hurl back retaliatory points, such as:

'You gave Janet time off.'
'I wasn't the only one involved.'
'You didn't say anything to so-and-so when they did the same thing.'

It's very easy to get drawn into an argument or discussion which takes you away from the point you want to make. What you need to do is have ready a very clear statement of the message you want to get across:

'I want a guarantee that the same thing won't happen again.'
'We need to talk about what happened at the meeting.'
'I wish to speak to the person in charge.'

Once you have got your phrase ready, use it when you need to stick to the point of the conversation. You may need to repeat your message, but don't just ignore what the other person says. Do this with a broad phrase which shows that you have heard what has been said, but which does not pick up and follow the content. Try a phrase like:

'That might be the case, but [repeat core phrase].'
'We can discuss that later. For now, [repeat core phrase].'

Speaking in the right way

Before you speak, take a few deep breaths and relax your muscles. This will help you to feel calm and grounded, and will help you to control your voice so that it doesn't sound whiney or squeaky or too abrupt. What you are aiming for is a tone of voice which matches the emotion you're communicating. Your voice should be firm, clear and animated. Try to hit medium volume. If you speak too softly you will sound nervous or unconvincing, and speaking too loudly will make you appear aggressive. Don't try to mask your emotion, though. Controlled doesn't mean lacking in feeling. Speaking at a pace and with a tone which show that you are worked up about the situation will help you to communicate your anger more effectively. If you feel passionate, speak passionately. Raise your voice when you are engaged and excited about what you are saying – just be careful not to shout at anyone.

Making your body language fit your words

Don't come across as weak

Your message will be diminished or even destroyed if your facial expression and your gestures indicate nervousness or lack of conviction. Smiling when you are angry suggests that you want to lessen the impact of your words, and gives the impression that you are anxious to please even though you are expressing displeasure. If you avoid eye contact you will seem awkward and unconvincing. Be careful with your gestures. If you cross your arms in front of your body you will seem to be on the defensive, and clasping your hands together may indicate nerves and tension. Touching your face can look nervous as well.

Don't come across as aggressive

If your assertive words are accompanied by punchy non-verbal language you will be perceived as aggressive, despite what you actually say. Try to ensure that you don't grimace or scowl too heavily, and don't stare the other person down. Control your posture and your gestures – don't loom over the other person, or stand too close to them. Be careful not to make jabbing or pointing movements with your hands and fingers.

How to support your words with appropriate body language

Your non-verbal messages should underline the seriousness of your message. Your body language should be forceful but controlled, and be consistent with what you are saying.

Posture

Go for alert, upright posture, whether you are standing or sitting down. If you are seated, lean forward slightly to convey a sense of urgency. It's best to be on the same level as the person you are talking to.

Gestures

Keep your gestures open. Have your hands in a palms-upward position, and if you need to add force to your words, put your hands a little apart with the palms facing inwards. Bringing both your hands down as you speak will add emphasis to what you say and will lead you to bring your voice down as well, which will give your words authority and prevent any tendency to sound squeaky or upset. If you want to communicate depth of feeling, use large, sweeping hand and arm gestures.

Facial expression

You want to look as if you mean what you are saying. No matter how nervous you feel, don't smile. Let your expression mirror your feelings – you will probably frown as you speak, or look very serious. As you are speaking, look the person in the eyes, but glance away now and then to avoid going into staring mode. If you glance down, do so as you speak, not after you have spoken, and look up again quickly. This will stop any impression that you are feeling intimidated.

Developing empathy

Empathy describes the ability to step into someone else's skin and experience the situation as if you were that person. It's what happens when you look at things from someone else's point of view and tune in to the emotions that he or she is experiencing. Responding empathetically to someone is particularly challenging when you seem to be on opposite sides, as is usually the case when you're angry. When anger engulfs us it is very difficult to see outside ourselves and our own needs and recognize and experience our antagonist's feelings. But when you learn to do this, you will find that your anger becomes less sharp and fierce, and that when you genuinely tune in to someone's emotional state, and don't just pay lip service to it, you are beginning the process of true communication and understanding which is the way to peaceful co-existence.

When we are feeling angry with someone, our instinctive response can be to accuse, criticize or judge the other person. We see that we are in the right and they are in the wrong, and our main concern is to express how angry we are and let them know just how out of order their behaviour is.

An empathetic response doesn't diminish the wrong that has been done, or look for excuses for behaviour that has hurt us. It doesn't mean that you hold back from expressing your anger for fear of offending someone. What it does mean is that you feel and show sensitivity to whatever feelings the other person has, and that you can get a hold on their view of the situation. Entering another person's world is a huge step, with huge benefits:

- You feel less hostile.
- You are aware of the other person as a fallible human being, who has needs and faults just as you do.
- You can prevent your anger from rising.
- You can begin to focus on a situation to be dealt with or a problem to be solved, rather than on a person who is making you angry.

How to develop empathy

When you're having a conversation with someone, ask yourself what that person is thinking and how that person is feeling. One very powerful way to experience how someone else is feeling is to look carefully at their body language. Don't limit this just to people in angry or distressed states – notice as much as you can about the facial expressions, gestures, postures and tone of voice that accompany different moods and states of mind. Then, in private, practise the same body language. Stand or sit in the same way, assume the same expression. You will find that this helps you to experience how the other person feels.

Another thing to practise is using an empathetic voice. This means speaking at the same sort of pitch and pace as the other person, and using the same kinds of words. Our vocal patterns reveal a lot about our feelings and the way we see ourselves and the world, and experiencing how someone communicates gives you an insight into their point of view.

Tuning in

Ruth is listening to her colleague Jamie describe his visit to one of their difficult clients, which he says in the end went all right and presented no cause for concern. There is no need to visit the family again. Ruth listens to his words and also observes his body language and the way that he speaks. In private, when the conversation is over and she is thinking about how to proceed, she sits on the edge of her chair as Jamie did, and leans forward with her shoulders hunched and her neck stiff. She can feel enormous tension in her body. She repeats his words, using the same tone and delivery style: 'It was okay' – pause – 'I mean, there was nothing specific' – pause – 'nothing to worry us' – pause – 'really.' Ruth can feel the uncertainty as the words are almost forced out, and this exercise confirms her previous observation that the visit was more worrying than Jamie is admitting, and that although he doesn't want to admit it, he is not as confident about the situation as he claims to be. She will talk to him again about it.

Ruth's empathetic skills enable her to pick up someone's state of mind without being challenging or confrontational. This approach is of great benefit to her in both her professional and her personal life.

Exercise 6.1: Developing your empathetic skills

Use this exercise for observation and practice to help you develop your empathetic skills.

1 Jot down the name of the person you observed, and briefly describe

their posture, gestures, facial expression, tone of voice and the feelings you picked up.

2 Put yourself into the position described and speak a few words in the same way.

3 Note what feelings you experienced.

Person _____

Posture _____

Gestures _____

Face _____

Tone _____

Feelings _____

My feelings _____

Developing listening skills

Angry situations become worse when we don't listen to each other. When we have rows, arguments, altercations, we may hear the words that the other person speaks but often we don't really attend to them. We get the gist of what is being said and respond accordingly, or we pick up only the words that we want to hear. We don't get the whole message: we get the parts of it that fit in with our view of the situation and that justify the position we are taking. We interrupt, we contradict, we disagree, we fight back, we have an overriding urge to make our point regardless of what the other person is saying.

Active listening is a crucial communication skill, and it's one which demands a lot from us, even in friendly conversations. It is even more difficult to apply when we are angry and het up, but these are the circumstances in which active listening can play a highly valuable role in helping us to manage the conflict and move towards a resolution.

Try to practise the following key skills in undemanding situations, so that you become used to this way of responding and will be more able to use them easily.

Attending

We don't always pay full attention to what someone is saying to us. We are half tuned in, but at the same time we are thinking about what we are going to say next, or we are concentrating on our own feelings. Listening actively means being prepared to move outside yourself and, as the other person speaks, put your own needs and preoccupations on hold.

Try to listen to the other person using more than just your ears. If you use your ears only, it is likely that you will hear only the top layer of the message. Engage your empathetic skills to help you take in the whole of the message that is coming across. Listen with your body as well – be aware of the other person's body language, and show by your non-verbal communication that you are giving your whole attention to what is being said.

Do:

- Nod and make head movements to show that you are hearing what is being said. (This is not the same as agreeing with it.)
- Maintain eye contact.
- Keep your gestures open.
- Sit or stand in the same kind of position as the other person.

Don't:

- Interrupt.
- Look down or away.
- Do something else at the same time.
- Shake your head in disagreement.
- Speak at a different volume and pace from the other person.

Reflecting

This means that you listen with empathy to what the other person is saying, and feed back what you have heard in a way that reflects both the content and the emotion of what has been said:

> 'So you're having a go at me because you think that I spent too much on the new kitchen.'

'You're angry because I said you couldn't sleep over at Frankie's house again.'
'You feel that I didn't consider your position when I organized the restructure.'
'You were so busy today that you completely forgot that we'd arranged to go out.'

The simple act of reflecting what you have heard lowers the temperature of an argument and makes the other person less defensive. It also increases your understanding of their emotional state and helps you to continue the conversation calmly. One of the advantages of this approach is that it helps you to keep track of the issue, because you keep checking that you have heard correctly and that you have understood. This gives both people involved an opportunity to clear up misunderstandings before they escalate.

Keeping an open mind

A very challenging aspect of listening is putting aside our prejudices and preconceptions, and attending with an open mind. Often we make assumptions, and hear what we want to hear or expect to hear. Try to focus all your attention on exactly what the other person is saying, and be aware of their non-verbal signals as well as their words. Don't get distracted by your own thoughts and judgements.

Asking clarifying questions

One of the main purposes of listening is to understand what is going on with the other person. Asking helpful questions is a way of getting more information and more insight into someone's position. It also demonstrates your focus on the other person, which indicates that you are prepared to pay attention to their needs as well as your own.

Some useful questions include:

'Tell me some more about …'
'Is there anything else I should know?'
'Can you tell me exactly what you mean by that?'
'What can we do to make this better?'
'What would you like to happen?'

Communicating when an angry outburst takes you by surprise

Being at the receiving end of an explosion of anger is a disturbing and frightening experience, and the force of the emotion can seem like a battering ram coming straight at you. Whether the anger is justified or not does not matter at this point. The point is that the person who is angry is in a highly aroused emotional state and is not able to think or behave rationally. The anger is their problem and responsibility, not yours. You are responsible for managing your own feelings and reactions. Be aware that the way that you respond can help the situation or make it worse. What you need to do is behave in a way that is likely to take the heat out of the situation and create a calmer atmosphere. Only when this is established will you be able to communicate about whatever the issue is. Attempting at first to do anything else – defend yourself, ask questions, have a reasonable discussion – is doomed to failure because the other person is not able at the moment to exercise judgement or control.

Get in the right mode

Tell yourself that you are moving into 'anger management' mode. Your instinctive, automatic response to face-to-face anger may always have been to fight your corner and shout back, or you may have a pattern of shrinking and being intimidated by the other person. You don't need to resort to these behaviours. It may take some time to get used to managing hostility positively, but with practice you will become used to it.

Control your physical reactions

The first thing you need to do is deal with the automatic 'fight or flight' response which kicks in. You can short-circuit this response by switching into a state which is both relaxed and ready for appropriate action. Try to find an equilibrium of calm and alertness. You don't want to appear angry yourself, nor do you want to give the impression that you are scared or avoiding the issue. Take one or two deep breaths as described on p. 101. Check that your body hasn't tensed for an aggressive response – if your hands have flown into fists, let them hang loose; if your shoulders are hunched and clenched, let them drop.

The angry person will pick up any aggressive signals you send, and is likely to become more angry and aggressive. Move into a position where you do not communicate a sense of threat. Don't stand face to face, which will give the impression that you are squaring up for a fight, and try to get on the same level as the other person. Don't tower over someone, or let them tower over you, and keep a comfortable space between you. Make sure that you both have access to an exit – don't block a doorway, or allow someone else to block it. Even if it is not the kind of situation in which you need to get out, you still want to create a feeling of co-operation and safety. If the incident is occurring at work or in a public place and you feel that you need to get the person to go somewhere else, as you start to talk move in the direction you want to take, indicating the way with your arm pointing and your palm open and facing the person, as if you are accompanying them. Sometimes a change of venue is a good idea anyway, as it breaks the momentum of the emotional outburst.

Use a coping statement such as:

'I won't let this anger infect me.'
'There is no need for me to get angry.'
'This is a situation that we can sort out.'

Watch what you say

What you need to do is acknowledge the other person's anger. She is unlikely to take in any details of what you say at this point, but will respond to the tone of your voice and to words which show that you are tuned in to her feelings. An empathetic statement such as:

'I can see how much this has got to you,'
'I understand that you're very angry,'
'You're really upset about this,'

indicates validation of the other person's feelings without being patronizing or diminishing his or her emotion. This is not the time to say anything like 'Calm down' or 'We can't talk about this while you're shouting at me.' That kind of comment is likely to cause antagonism and make things worse.

You can make it clear that you understand the person's message without condoning or arguing against the reasons for the anger. Saying 'I can hear how angry you are' is not the same as saying that you think the person's feelings are justified. When someone feels that her feelings are acknowledged, she doesn't need to continue demonstrating them so intensely, and there is likely to be a softening effect which will prevent the anger from escalating.

Get the right tone and pace

If you speak very quietly and calmly, you are likely to have the opposite effect to the one that you want. This tone can make you seem removed and detached and as if you actually don't understand the nature of the person's feelings. It can make you sound patronizing and can be quite inflammatory. On the other hand, you don't want to speak as forcefully and angrily as the other person. A good strategy is to begin speaking almost as intensely as the other, and just under the same pitch. Then you gradually lower your voice and speak more slowly as you engage in a dialogue. Keep the pace slow and even and make your gestures controlled and relaxed.

Disclose your feelings

If you are feeling uncomfortable or are getting upset, it's fine to acknowledge this if you think it's appropriate. Be careful to take responsibility for your own feelings and not to blame the other person for your reaction.

Don't say: 'You're making me feel nervous.'
Say: 'I'm feeling nervous because you are shouting.'

Listen and reflect

Show that you are listening to what is being said. As soon as you sense that the anger is subsiding sufficiently for the person to hear your words, reflect back what you have understood.

'You're furious because I forgot to renew the insurance.'
'You're angry because you feel I embarrassed you in front of your friends.'
'You're angry because the report I prepared wasn't detailed enough.'

Make it clear that you want to discuss the problem and find a solution:

> 'We really need to talk about this, when we are both feeling calm.'
> 'I can see why you're so annoyed. I want to do something to help.'
> 'I'd like to find a way of sorting this out.'

Take time

You might need to postpone discussion until you can communicate as calmly as is necessary. Depending on the circumstances, say something like:

> 'We need to sort this out. Shall we get together after the meeting?'
> 'Let's give it half an hour and talk about it then.'
> 'You've brought up a lot of stuff that I need to think about. Let's talk about it tomorrow when we've got the house to ourselves.'

Nipping an angry outburst in the bud

If you respond quickly you might be able to prevent the storm that is brewing. You need to be able to intervene while the person is still in a position to respond rationally to what you say, or at least to hear it. You might be able to recognize the signs that someone's anger levels are rising. People's facial expressions can indicate imminent fury, as can their gestures and posture. You might notice patterns of behaviour which suggest that sooner or later there is going to be an explosion, perhaps a series of little verbal digs, growing lack of co-operation, grumpiness or sulkiness.

Try showing that you realize the other person is getting wound up. You could say: 'There seems to be something on your mind' or 'Something's bothering you. Like to talk about it?' or 'Have I done something to annoy you?' Of course, this might precipitate an angry outburst, but you won't be taken by surprise. You have initiated the conversation and will be in a good position to control your responses and manage the situation.

If you feel intimidated or in physical danger

You don't have to tolerate being shouted at. Don't shout back, but say very firmly that you are not continuing the discussion. Say, 'You are shouting at me, and I'm going to walk away.'

Ask for help if you have the slightest feeling that you need to. You don't need to sound alarmed. For example, at work, say something like, 'I think John could help us with this. I'm going to buzz him.'

If someone shows signs of physical aggression, don't hesitate to leave.

Don't meet violence with violence.

If your work means that you often encounter angry or potentially violent clients or customers, make sure that you are familiar with the safety and support procedures that are in place, and be confident about using them when required.

If you experience violence at home, contact one of the organizations which exist to help people in your situation. You will find some suggestions in the Useful addresses section (p. 131).

Communicating when anger is hidden

At least you know where you are when someone confronts you with an outburst of anger. Far more insidious are the expressions of anger which are covert or indirect, when people clam up and won't say what is bothering them, or behave in ways which indicate pent-up emotion while proclaiming that there is nothing wrong.

Recognize the signs

With family and people close to you, you can learn to recognize the signs that someone is harbouring anger or resentment. They may retreat into themselves, or become monosyllabic, or have certain behaviour patterns that come into play – stomping around aggressively, or engaging in vigorous cleaning of the car or the kitchen, or throwing themselves into work, or becoming critical of insignificant things. With some work colleagues you may be able to spot the same signs. Look out for any incidents where someone seems to be sabotaging you in some way – claiming not to have received stuff you have sent, making disparaging remarks, not passing on messages. This kind of behaviour may be the person's way of expressing anger.

Open it up

You might feel it's not worth saying anything because the other person won't admit that anything is up, but ignoring the behaviour and what it implies is not going to solve the situation. And after all, if people really want to keep their feelings to themselves they find ways of doing so.

The most positive way to approach this situation is to indicate that you know something is wrong:

'What's bothering you?'
'Something's up – what is it?'
'Are you angry with me about something?'

If you get a negative reply, push it a little further, being careful not to blame or accuse:

'I'm asking because you've been very quiet these past few evenings.'
'It's just that you've locked yourself in the study.'
'It's unlike you not to finish your favourite meal.'
'You seemed annoyed that the children were playing video games, but that doesn't usually bother you.'
'You have been offhand with me ever since I spoke out at the meeting.'
'I've noticed that you don't phone me as you used to.'

Be prepared to be specific, and try to give examples from more than one context.

Don't say: 'You've been having a go at me all week.'
Say: 'You snapped at me when I got back from the gym, and you were really annoyed when I forgot to cancel the milk.'

Discover the source of the anger

You may have to dig a little and encourage the other person to be precise about what has got to him or her. This might involve you presenting your interpretation of the situation:

'I was wondering if you were angry because I invited Bill and Orla over at the weekend.'
'It seems to me that you might still be annoyed because I wouldn't give you a lift to town the other day.'
'I get the impression that you're not happy with some of the decisions I've made.'

To get to the precise point, you may need to instigate specific criticism of your behaviour.

'So do you think that I was thoughtless?'
'Did I not listen carefully enough to what you said?'
'Can you give me an example of when I was rude to your friends?'

Move it on

Once the anger and its cause are out in the open, you can show that you want to discuss ways of making things better, or if this is not possible at the moment, you can indicate your appreciation that the air has been cleared.

'What can I do differently?'
'Would it help us both if ...?'
'Thanks for letting me know how you feel.'

7

Handling hostile personal situations

Some relationships seem to thrive on rows. There are couples who have regular screaming matches accompanied by plate-throwing and storming out, and claim that it is worth it for the making-up. There are families whose main mode of communication is through rows and aggression. Others boast that they haven't had a cross word in years. Neither extreme is a good model for healthy co-existence. Destructive anger ruins lives, and so does anger which is repressed and buried. Managing angry feelings and communicating them in an effective and non-confrontational way is the best way of handling the rows and disagreements which, if mismanaged, can cause distress and havoc in our lives.

The nature of personal rows

With people we are close to, our emotions are heightened, and there is a lot at stake. If you get in a temper with a colleague or with someone in a call centre or with an unhelpful shop assistant, the context of the row gives it boundaries, and your anger is likely to be over quickly. Have you ever heard it said that someone 'never got over the argument she had with the travel company about getting a refund for her holiday – she hasn't been the same since'? Yet all too often we hear about people who 'never got over' a family row at Christmas which has left some members not speaking to each other years later, and about close friends whose falling out over something seemingly trivial means that the friendship is finished or permanently damaged.

In rows with partners, family, friends, those who mean a lot to us, we are sometimes more extreme in what we say. We go further than we would with people who are more distant from us. We don't hold back, and we fight dirty. There is the unspoken assumption that we are more forgiving with those we love and that hurtful and damaging speech and behaviour will be easily forgotten.

What do you argue about?

The range of things that cause arguments is huge. Because of the way that the different lives and expectations of men and women have evolved over recent years, there is less clear demarcation of roles and responsibilities and more grounds for conflict and strife. Some of the common triggers for rows include:

- allocation of domestic chores and duties;
- how money is spent;
- how to deal with children;
- how time is spent;
- work intruding on home life;
- comparative importance attributed to each one's job;
- decisions about the house, holidays, etc.;
- disrespectful behaviour;
- feeling let down;
- being lied to or cheated on;
- being criticized;
- being put down or diminished;
- sex.

Add your own ideas:

_____

_____

_____

Exercise 7.1: Finding a pattern

See if there is a pattern in the things that get you riled. Identify the people and the issues involved.

	Person	Situation	How I feel
1			
2			
3			
4			

What do you really argue about?

Often the presenting cause of dispute is not the real reason for anger. We argue about money or household matters, and what's actually getting to us could be something else entirely. It could be that we feel neglected, or inadequate, or helpless. When our basic needs for security, affection, attention, recognition, control are thwarted, we feel angry and frustrated, and if we can't express this need we make our feelings known in other ways.

It could be that arguments bring up memories of other hostile encounters, or incidents that happened ages ago. Maybe the way that your family handled anger and confrontation is evoked, and this memory influences the way that you handle angry feelings now. Or it could be that every argument reminds you of how you or the other person acted the last time, or during a significant exchange some time ago. In these cases your focus isn't on the here and now. You are responding to an old situation.

Who are you really arguing with?

Often we take out our anger on people who aren't its cause. You have a row at work which leaves you feeling punchy and jittery, so you argue that evening about whose turn it is to pick the kids up from swimming; you're furious with your brother for assuming that you will take your elderly father to a hospital appointment, so you turn on your son for waking you up when he comes home late.

If you find yourself firing up at someone when your reaction is out of proportion to the situation, stop and check who you are really angry with. Decide if you need to express your anger and open a discussion with that person.

How to have a good argument

A good row isn't one which just enables you to let off steam and bring your feelings out into the open – that may relieve your tension, but it is not positive. A good row is one which results in deeper understanding, more tolerance and a determination to keep a sense of perspective and an awareness of what each values in the other.

Your argument stands a chance of being clear, focused and non-damaging if from the start you both know what you're arguing about and you are both arguing about the same thing. There also needs to be an intention to get a better situation as a result of your dialogue.

The following suggestions extend the previous chapter's guidelines for expressing your feelings assertively, and offer some ideas for how to make sure that your relationships are enhanced and not damaged by the exchange of strong feelings.

Stay focused

Be clear about:

- the issue that you are angry about;
- how you feel;
- what you would like to happen.

Get the right time and place

Have you noticed how some people choose to instigate an argument or a difficult conversation just as you're rushing to get out of the door on time, or when you're on your way to an evening out with friends, or when you're settling down to watch the DVD you've been looking forward to all day? If you are going to have a productive discussion it needs to take place at a time when you can both give it full attention, and in a place where there is sufficient privacy for you to speak freely and openly. If something flares up at an inappropriate time, it's best not to follow it up but to agree to talk about it later.

Some people like to choose 'neutral' territory for this kind of conversation, and opt for talking over a meal or a drink in a bar or pub. A disadvantage is that this may give a falsely social air to the conversation, and another disadvantage is that it might not be wise to drink even a little alcohol when the conversation may get heated or confrontational.

Make a clear statement about why you are angry

Own and express your feelings. Be precise and specific about the behaviour that you are reacting to.

Don't say: 'I'm angry with the way you treated me last night.'

Say: 'I'm angry because you ignored my statement that I wanted to go home in the next half hour.'

Don't say: 'I'm disappointed that you are being so stupid.'

Say: 'I'm angry because you have started smoking.'

Don't say: 'You're so thoughtless.'

Say: 'I get really annoyed when you don't tell me that you're going to be late home.'

Stick to the here and now

In the heat of the moment, you may well think of all the other times when the person has done things that have upset you. Don't bring them up. When you say things like, 'What about the time when ...' or 'This is exactly what you did last year,' you drift off the point and revisit old grievances rather than focus on the present.

When someone does this to you, say: 'Let's just talk about what happened today.'

Stick to the specific

In the heat of the moment, it's very easy to generalize:

'That's typical of you.'
'You always say that.'
'You can never be trusted.'
'You always complain.'
'You only ever think of yourself.'

These comments usually burst out when you're frustrated and feel that you're getting nowhere. When you say something like this you are moving away from the issue at stake and launching a character attack, and you probably expect to provoke an angry defence or counter-attack. The best thing to do, when this remark is about to fly out of your mouth, is just not say it. Instead, repeat the specific thing that you're complaining about.

When someone does this to you, don't get drawn in, and on no account turn the generalized comment into another thread of the argument: 'Oh, so now it's that I can never be trusted, is it? Well, if we're speaking about trust ...' You can defuse the situation by gently challenging the generalization with something like: 'There must be the odd time when you can trust me, surely?' or 'Oh, I can think of the odd occasion when I haven't complained.'

If you want to acknowledge that there's some truth in the gist of the accusation, say something like, 'You're right, I am selfish sometimes. But I don't think I was on this occasion,' or 'You're right, I did behave selfishly. But you know, my behaviour isn't always like that.'

Don't interrupt

Even if what's being said seems so unreasonable or out of order or mistaken that you feel you can't let the person continue, don't burst in and say so. Remember your listening skills. What you need to do is listen and empathize, then reply. Don't just wait for the other person to draw breath so that you can dive in with what you were going to say anyway.

If you are interrupted, say something like, 'Let's agree to hear each other out.'

Don't blame

When things go wrong and you become angry, your instinct can be to blame the other person:

'You've ruined the whole evening!'
'It's your fault for forgetting the keys.'
'It would have been all right if you hadn't opened your big mouth.'

Blame is accusatory and its only purpose is to make the other person feel bad. Whatever happened may well be the other person's fault, but by hurling blame you do nothing to make the situation any better and may well succeed in making it worse. When you blame you indicate that you are not interested in listening or in focusing on the problem. You have decided where the fault lies and you are giving the definitive ruling on the situation.

If you are blamed, there are a couple of ways to respond. If you really are at fault and this is the only possible view of the situation, take it on the chin. Admit your responsibility and apologize. Then focus on the problem, and say how you feel about the other person's anger: 'In future, we need to work out a way of making sure we have the keys. I don't like you being so angry with me,' or, if you feel there are other issues here: 'Is there anything else that's making you angry?'

If the situation is not quite as cut and dried – and this is usually the case – own up to your part and perhaps try some humour: 'I realize I didn't help the evening by disappearing into the kitchen so that Andrea could cry on my shoulder, but hey, I think their weird décor/cooking/choice of music/unruly pets affected everyone badly.'

Don't counter-attack

It's a defensive mechanism to shoot back with a 'what about you' barb, a natural instinct but not a helpful one. When we do this we are just hitting out blindly instead of listening and responding to what is being said.

When someone does this to you, say something like: 'Yes, I know I've been critical of some of the men in your life, but at the moment, I'm saying that I don't like the way you criticize Greg.'

Don't give ultimatums

Ultimatums can be very dramatic and can give a real punch to your message, but unless you really, really mean what you say, don't deliver them.

Don't say things deliberately to hurt

Your intimate knowledge of someone close to you gives you a range of weapons that you could use in a fight. At work also, there may be colleagues who you know well enough to have a pretty good idea of what makes them tick. In these cases, you know which buttons to push. Tempting though it may be in the heat of the moment, don't do it.

Protect yourself from hurtful remarks

Other people, of course, may play dirty, so be on the alert for it. Being aware of your vulnerable points will help you to have in place some protective strategies when people attack these particular areas. Identify the individuals and activities and ideas that really matter to you, perhaps because they are the aspects of your life in which you invest most of yourself, or because they are areas that you would like to be a lot better, or they are areas which matter to you a lot but in which you feel that you fail. The areas in which we take most pride, or by which we define ourselves, are the ones in which we can be easily hurt. Be ready for the jolt and the defensive kick you will experience when someone makes a jibe about these aspects, and be prepared to manage your reaction.

Points of pride

Laurie is a pretty average driver. She is safe and steady behind the wheel and prefers to drive comparatively slowly. She's not very confident or indeed very skilful, as the odd bump and scrape testify, and she finds motorway driving particularly taxing. Laurie knows this and doesn't care at all. When people mock her reluctance to overtake or the fact that she takes ages to park in a tight spot she just laughs.

Laila, on the other hand, prides herself on being a fast confident driver who has never had an accident. Her partner knows that all it takes is a dig at Laila's driving to really get her upset.

Jayne has a thing about maintaining a spotless home. All it takes is a reference to something not being clean or tidy and she gets very hurt and defensive. With Roxy, it's her job as a nurse. Any suggestion that she has failed in the quality of care that she gives hits her like a blow in the stomach.

The way to protect yourself is to have ready a statement you can say to yourself that helps you to keep calm:

'I know I'm a good driver. I will just ignore this comment.'
'I know I keep the house clean. If there is the occasional slip-up, it's not the end of the world. I won't let this get to me.'
'I know I'm a good nurse. Sometimes things won't be as I'd like them to be. I always give my best. This comment won't damage me.'

Then if you wish you can say to the other person something like:

'I'm not going to respond to that.'

You could add, depending on the type and stage of the argument:

'I think you said that just to hurt me. It's got nothing to do with what we're talking about.'

Exercise 7.2: Protecting your pride

What do you pride yourself on? Choose three areas. Work out what you will say if these buttons are pushed.

	Area	What I will say to myself	What I will reply
1			
2			
3			

Areas of guilt

Rosina feels guilty because she isn't always able to go to school events like plays and concerts. It's very difficult for her to get time off for events held during working hours, and she prefers to keep days in hand for emergencies like sickness. She feels rotten when people talk about what she missed and say what a shame that she didn't see Harry bringing down the house as the inn-keeper.

Jill feels guilty because her mother lives in a care home and Jill blames herself for not being able to give her mother a home with her and her family. Megan feels guilty because she wishes that her grown-up children would leave home. Irish feels guilty because she doesn't like her step-daughter.

The best way to protect yourself in these areas is to get rid of the guilt, or at least make it manageable:

'I would like to go to all school events, but I can't. That doesn't make me a bad mother.'

'I am doing the best I can for my mother. There is no point feeling bad about things I can't do.'

'I love my children, and I wish they would find homes of their own.'

'It's all right not to find everyone likeable. I can still have a civil relationship with Chloe.'

Then you will be ready to say something like:

'I'm not rising to that one.'

You could add, depending on the type and stage of the argument:

'I think you said that to make me feel bad. It's got nothing to do with what we're talking about.'

Exercise 7.3: What do you feel guilty about?

Yes, it's difficult not to answer 'everything'. But choose three areas that are closest to home and in which you are most vulnerable and work out what you will say if these buttons are pushed.

	Area	What I will say to myself	What I will reply
1			
2			
3			

Don't demean or put down

Other ways of inflicting hurt are to speak with contempt, or sneer at the other person. If you do this, you show that you are not interested in communicating and finding a resolution, but that your intention is to demean and humiliate.

If you are put down, say something like:

'That's very hurtful. You probably didn't mean it to be.'

Don't play psychologist

It's not helpful to imply that you know a person better than they know themselves. Playing this card in an argument suggests that you think you are superior to the other person, and also indicates that you are not prepared to listen because you have already decided what makes them tick. Avoid saying things like: 'You're insecure because your parents split up when you were young' or 'You've got a power complex.'

Be ready to walk away

If you feel that either of you is losing control, and that things may be said which will be regretted later, take time out. You might need just ten minutes or so, or you might need to put the discussion on hold until another appropriate time. Make clear that this is what you are doing, and that the conversation isn't over, just postponed.

Absolutely no physical violence

Don't inflict it and don't take it. If you follow the above suggestion, it shouldn't be a problem.

Try humour

It depends on the circumstances and on your relationship, but the ability to step outside what is going on for just a minute and find something to laugh at really does take the heat out of the moment. A touch of deliberate exaggeration, a bit of self-deprecation, a reference to an experience you have shared or a comparison of yourselves to television or film characters you both know can all do the trick. Just be careful not to seem as if you are laughing at someone or mocking their feelings.

Words that work and words that don't

Some killer phrases to avoid

- 'The trouble with you is ...'
- 'There's no point in talking to you ...'
- 'And another thing ...'

Add your own ideas (be honest, you probably have some of your own favourites ...):

_____

_____

_____

Some winning phrases to use

- 'What can I do to make this better?'
- 'I'm sorry.'

Add your own ideas:

_____

_____

_____

Change your perspective

Live with differences

There is no reason why anybody else, even your spouse or partner or your best friend, should share your tastes, interests, attitudes or values. Relationships can flourish in spite of differences ranging from choices of holiday destinations to supporting different political parties or belonging to different religious groups. If differences are a cause of anger, go for negotiation and agreement to build on your similarities. Focus on what draws you together, and find interest and stimulus in the areas in which you differ.

Don't hang on

Sometimes we hang on to relationships which are dead in the water. In some of these cases we focus so much on dealing with the anger and hostility that we lose sight of the overall picture. If all you do is argue and if every argument confirms that there is little care or respect for each other or that one person just wants to inflict pain and hurt on the other, and you are unable to move beyond this situation, then you could think about seeking expert help to enable you to make decisions about the relationship.

Turning conflict into co-operation

Get the right focus

When anger has been aired and has subsided, you can build on the knowledge and insight you have gained to help you resolve the conflict. You make a transition from the stage of the argument in which each of you seeks to score points off the other as you both vie for the upper hand, and begin to look at the problem itself. You focus on the core of the issue, without being concerned about who is in the right and who is in the wrong. Instead of arguing about who left the kitchen in a mess and why you've run out of milk again, focus on how best to organize the household. Rather than quarrel about the amount of time someone spends playing golf, or going shopping, or seeing family members, focus on how best to use your spare time. Rather than take up opposing sides on decisions about your children's education, focus on exploring the options which might best meet their needs and interests. Research conducted over a period of twenty years by the American psychologist John Gottman identifies the ability to solve conflict as one of the defining features of a successful marriage – and the skills required for achieving this may be put to good use in every area of your life.

Understand each other's feelings and point of view

Key skills to use here are listening and empathizing. Tune in to the other person or persons involved. Identify what their needs are, and check your understanding by reflecting back to them what has come across to you.

Open questions are helpful here:

'Tell me why you think we shouldn't go ahead with the garage conversion.'
'What do you think might happen if we tell Amelia that we're not willing to fund her holiday?'

Hypothetical questions are a good way to develop the discussion further:

'What's the worst thing that could happen if we agreed to...?'
'Suppose we did ...'
'Just imagine for a moment that we ...'

This type of question presents a gentle and unthreatening way of exploring difficult topics, and of discovering more about somebody's thoughts and feelings on the issue.

Find common grounds and interests

This is the key to handling conflict in a collaborative way. You look for solutions that will go some way to satisfying the needs of everyone involved, so that no one feels a winner at someone else's expense, and no one feels a loser whose wishes haven't been met. Exploring this option takes perseverance, a desire to make it work, and a willingness not to hang on to your original position.

Focusing on needs rather than on the solution you have already identified is crucial to this process. If you both 'need' the only car at the same time, the 'need' is actually to get to a certain place. You can think of other ways of meeting this need.

Adopting a collaborative and problem-solving approach

Taking a proactive approach to our worries and concerns helps us to feel calm and in control. Even difficult and challenging situations need not turn into overwhelming catastrophes or develop into anger and hostility. You can apply problem-solving strategies to issues which confront you, and in the course of tackling difficulties in this proactive and positive way, you will discover more about yourself and learn and develop new skills.

> *The family holiday*
> Tempers are getting very frayed in Sarah's household. They are trying to arrange a holiday which will suit Sarah and James, their teenage daughter plus her friend, and their younger son. What should be an enjoyable task is turning into one huge row. Sarah is getting angry because she feels that her need for a bit of rest and relaxation is not being recognized, and that no one understands that she doesn't like too much heat. Holly and her friend think that Sarah just wants to go somewhere with no life, and that no one understands that all they want is sun and clubbing. Toby is sulking because he thinks Holly will get whatever she wants. James is firing up because he thinks the children are being selfish.
>
> Sarah decides to approach this problem calmly and systematically to see if they can generate a solution.

1 Define what the problem is

The first step in tackling a problem in an anger-free way is to define exactly what the issue is and what is causing the difficulty. Defining the problem as clearly as possible is a vital first step to dealing with it.

Instead of describing your problem as: 'I'm overweight', define it as: 'I want to lose x number of kilos.'

Another way to look at this is to identify the underlying need as well. Why do you want to lose weight? Do you need to be healthier, or to feel more attractive, or to fit into a particular outfit?

Instead of saying: 'I'm always broke', define it as: 'I need to have x amount more money every month.'

What's the underlying need here? Is it to be able to pay essential bills, or to maintain a certain lifestyle, or to feel you fit in with your group?

The more precisely you identify the problem, the easier it will be to find a solution.

Sarah decides that this issue is not only about deciding on a holiday destination, but about people feeling that their wishes and needs are being heard and acknowledged.

She defines the problem as:

What do we need to decide? Where to go on holiday.

What is getting in the way? Individual preferences, and people not listening to each other. People feeling that they are not being heard.

2 Decide what outcome you want

Decide what goal you are aiming for. Depending on the situation, there may be a single clear-cut goal, or there may be several strands that need to be addressed and incorporated. For a satisfactory outcome, the goal should be clearly and tangibly defined. You should be able to describe what you are aiming for in concrete terms, including the time-scale involved, and any other parameters such as cost or resources. Your goal description could include what you are or are not prepared to concede.

In Sarah's case, the necessary outcome is a decision about where they will go on holiday. She describes the goal as:

By 31 May, to have made a decision about where to go on holiday, with everyone feeling that they had a say in the process.

3 Generate options

This is the point at which you jot down all the ideas that occur to you. Let your mind roam free, and use this part of the process to address any additional and underlying challenges in the situation. The way in which you go about finding solutions to your problem can in itself decrease anger and tension. Including other people in the exercise, for example, and doing it as a joint activity may go some way to creating a more harmonious atmosphere. Put your instinct to evaluate ideas on hold – write everything down, no matter how far-fetched.

In Sarah's case, she needs to generate as many options and possibilities as she can to keep her mind open to all approaches, and she wants to include in her options suggestions which respect and include each person's voice and needs.

Sarah's list of options includes:

- Just decide on a place myself.
- Get James to decide on a place himself.
- We decide together and tell the kids that's what we're doing.
- Ask a friend to choose for us.
- Save arguments by not going away this year.
- Ask each person to identify their top priority requirement.
- Ask each person to be very precise about specific needs, e.g. need to be no more than x distance from beach/town, etc.
- Ask each person to identify the one thing they really don't want.
- Everyone comes up with three places that would suit them.
- Vote.
- Put all suggestions in hat and draw one out.
- Pick a place at random and hope for the best.

4 Assess the pros and cons of ideas

Now note the advantages and disadvantages of each option.

For example, one of the possibilities Sarah has identified is for her or James or the two of them together to make the decision. She notes about these options:

Advantages:
- Decision would be made quickly.
- We would both try to be fair.

Disadvantages:
- Others' resentment at not being consulted.
- They wouldn't feel involved.
- They might blame us or we might blame each other if anything went wrong.
- We may be being accused of favouritism in choice.

5 Make a choice

Choose the option or options that seem to you to have most going for them.

Sarah decides to bring everyone together and ask each of them to say in turn what are the two most important considerations for them. Everyone will then discuss what aspects people are prepared to compromise on. Then they will agree on three places that might fit the bill. Everyone chooses their favourite idea and writes it on a piece of paper. Then they come to a decision.

6 Identify the step or steps you need to take to get things started

Sarah decides to inform everyone that this is what will happen. She sets a date for a meal at home when they will discuss and decide the issue on the lines she has worked out.

This process helps Sarah feel less angry and aggrieved because her concerns are listened to, and the same goes for the others. The disagreements and arguments are channelled into a constructive approach to decision-making.

A problem-solving approach to situations that wind you up

The messy bedroom

Aisha gets wound up because her son's bedroom is always in a mess. She feels angry every time she goes past and sees the pile of clothes and stuff strewn everywhere, the collection of cups harbouring little cultures of penicillin, the dirty washing bursting out of the basket, the smell of shoes and socks ... Aisha knows it puts her in a bad mood, and it's beginning to get to her. She's tried yelling at him and making various threats, but nothing seems to work. It's actually spoiling their relationship because her son resents Aisha moaning at him all the time.

Aisha decides to approach this situation as a problem to be solved, not as a battle which she needs to win.

She begins by trying to define the issue. Is it that:

- she wants his room to be clean and tidy, and he doesn't?
- she wants not to feel angry about his messy room?
- she wants her son to do as she asks?
- she is worried about his room being a health hazard?
- she is angry because her son doesn't share her housekeeping standards?

- she feels embarrassed in case anyone else catches a glimpse of his room?

Aisha works out that the outcome she would like is for her to stay calm about the state of the room and not let it get to her.

She thinks of ways of achieving this goal. Ideas she comes up with include:

- putting the problem into perspective;
- using calming self-talk;
- asking her son to keep the door of his room closed so that she doesn't have to see it.

All these strategies, in fact, work for Aisha. She stays calm about the situation by telling herself: 'It's only a room. It's his own space. I can keep the rest of the house as I like. It's really not worth falling out over this.'

If this was your problem, you might see it differently, but you could apply the same process. For example, if your definition of the problem was that you wanted the room to be kept clean and tidy, you might generate solutions such as: speaking very assertively to your son; withdrawing a privilege or concession unless he does as you ask; compromising on the degree of tidiness required; locking him out of his room until he agrees to keep it clean; paying him to clean his room; agreeing that you will clean his room once a week.

Exercise 7.4: Problem-solving

Use this approach to help you solve a problem that is facing you at the moment.

Step 1
Define the problem

_____

_____

Step 2
Goals and outcomes

_____

_____

Step 3
All the possible options for dealing with the situation

_____

_____

Step 4
Advantages and disadvantages of the possible options

_____

_____

Step 5
Make a decision

_____

_____

Step 6
Action plan

_____

_____

Other ways of solving problems

- Think of things you haven't tried.
- Think of ridiculous possibilities, then ask yourself, 'Why not?'
- Ask a completely neutral person how he or she would approach it.
- Choose a role model for this purpose, someone who handles these situations effectively. What would this person do?

8

Taking charge of anger

Understanding and managing your moods

You may have noticed how the same event can arouse a different reaction, depending on the circumstances and your mood at the time. When you are feeling scratchy and grouchy something can grate on you and trigger your anger, whereas when you are feeling relaxed and mellow, your reaction may be entirely different.

Bev and the neighbours' barbecue

It's a hot summer's night and the people down the road are having a barbecue, their annual birthday celebration. The music and laughter and the smell of burgers on the grill drift through her open windows, and really get on her nerves. Bev is in a bad mood because she has had a blazing row with her husband and it has left her with a thumping headache. She bangs the window shut but it's too hot to keep it closed. They could spare a thought for other people, she thinks irritably, and resolves to glare at them next time they pass in the road.

The evening of last year's barbecue was also a hot one, and there had been the same mixture of noise and smells. But last year Bev was in a better frame of mind. She and Simon had enjoyed a day out with the children, and then they had chatted over a glass of wine in the garden. The sounds of the party down the road had seemed actually to reflect their good mood, and Bev had smiled tolerantly at the occasional extra-loud burst of music.

Recognizing and acknowledging the nature of your bad mood is the first step to dealing with it. Bev recognizes that she is in a grouchy mood because:

1 she is upset about the row;
2 she is physically uncomfortable – she has a headache and she's too hot.

It's not too difficult for her to deal with the physical complaints – she can ease the headache by taking a tablet, doing some relaxation exercises, going for a nap, going for a walk or applying whatever remedy usually works for her. She can take a cool shower and change her clothing.

She can calm herself down in the aftermath of the row by telling herself whatever is appropriate:

'It wasn't the end of the world – it was just a disagreement.'
'We can sort it out.'
'That was a bad row, and we can talk about the issues it brought up when we are both calm.'
'There is no point in projecting my anger with Simon on to the people down the road.'

These strategies help Bev to get into a better mood, and her feelings of anger about the barbecue do subside. She tells herself that after all it's only once a year, and no real harm is being done.

When you feel an angry and tetchy mood descending, use these kinds of self-talk and relaxation strategies to make you feel calmer and help you to respond more rationally to whatever is about to trigger or feed your anger. The better your frame of mind, the less likely you are to respond angrily to triggers and frustrations. When you're in a good mood, setbacks and annoyances can just bounce off you.

You might find it helpful to track any patterns that appear in your responses. There may be certain conditions that often make you react angrily. Are you always niggly when you're hungry, for example, or when you're in a hurry? Perhaps one of the ways that you realize you're tired and need to rest or go to bed is when you get snappy with people for no very good reason.

Exercise 8.1: What irritates you?

Make a note of occasions when you begin to feel irritated and annoyed without any significant provocation. Identify the physical context of these events. You could choose examples of context from these suggestions, or add your own.

Being hungry
Being dehydrated
Not having had enough sleep
Suffering from a headache
Being in pain

Being uncomfortable – tight shoes, etc.
Being in a rush
Feeling hemmed in
Feeling panicky
Feeling tense
Being too hot
Being too cold
Being a bit run down
Getting over an illness
Having something on your mind
Driving
Being a passenger in a car
Travelling on public transport
Being in a crowded shop
Dealing with heavy traffic
Trying to do several things at once
Children nagging you for something
Being on a diet
Giving up smoking
Longing for a cigarette
When you've had a few drinks
When you feel as if you want a drink
When you've got a hangover
Being in a noisy environment
When you're lost
Being in the presence of unpleasant smells
When it's raining
When it's January or February

Add your own examples:

	Occasion	Context	How I felt
1			
2			
3			
4			
5			
6			

When you recognize that certain situations are likely to trigger
feelings of anger, you can short-circuit the connection of events

by acknowledging what your mood is likely to be and taking some steps to prevent it.

Saturday at the DIY retail park

Abi is very happy with the plans she and Georgie have made for renovating the old house they have bought, and she is enjoying working on it at weekends. But whenever they have to make the Saturday or Sunday trip to buy the necessary tools and equipment, Abi finds herself getting tetchy and finding fault with everything. She snaps angrily when Georgie checks if they are sure about a certain colour paint for the hall, and flies off the handle when the store is out of the type of doorknob they want. This means that there are rows and tension every time they need to go through this process, so much so that they are both beginning to dread weekends.

Abi wonders what is making her behave like this. She examines her feelings to see if there is a hidden agenda. She is satisfied that she is not feeling any latent hostility to Georgie, and that she has no resentment about any aspect of this project they have undertaken – yet she seems to be sabotaging it. Eventually Abi realizes that she dislikes crowds and bustle, and this is why she hates going to the store. She dislikes the press of people, the way she has to manoeuvre past trolleys loaded with planks of wood and cans of paint and the way that people clog up the aisle deliberating about what to buy. Now she can make some choices, such as:

● Stop going to the store and letting Georgie do it alone.
● Find out the times that the store is likely to be least busy, and go then.
● Go to another town which has a smaller, less populated retail park.
● Manage her feelings of annoyance so that she can handle a short visit.

Life stages when anger may be more easily triggered

Women's lives are undoubtedly affected by hormonal activity, a fact which is sometimes used to dismiss female displays of hostility as the irrational outpourings of an unstable mind. Now and again, in extreme medical cases, this stereotype may have an element of truth, but on the whole it is an easy and lazy way of categorizing the complex processes that affect our bodies and our minds. We don't know for sure if fluctuating hormonal levels are the main reason for the moodiness and tetchiness many women feel at particular stages in their lives – other changes in the body's chemistry, personality, social factors may all be involved – but understanding how hormonal changes affect your behaviour is the first step to managing the anger, tension and irritability which you may experience in yourself and in others at certain stages.

Puberty and on

From the onset of puberty, hormones affect our bodies and our minds. As hormonal activity kicks in during the early and teenage years, it is common for young people of both genders to experience physical and emotional turbulence, often displayed in outbursts of anger and frustration.

Teenage tantrums

Rebecca wonders how her delightful young son has turned into this shouting, yelling, stroppy teenager. Everything Rebecca does or says is wrong: she's not fair, she doesn't understand, she never listens … It's as if Sam is on an emotional roller-coaster, up one minute, but you never know how long it will be before he plunges into the next bad mood. Today he stormed in, threw his school bag in the corner and stomped upstairs.

'What's wrong?' Rebecca called after him.

Sam muttered something unintelligible and slammed his door.

Rebecca works out a way of dealing with Sam's anger. She decides that she will wait until Sam is calmer, then:

- defuse the situation rather than complain about Sam's behaviour;
- acknowledge that Sam is feeling hostile and angry;
- give Sam an opportunity to talk about how he is feeling;
- not put pressure on Sam to talk if he doesn't want to;
- be clear about the kind of behaviour she won't accept;
- offer some suggestions about how Sam could manage his angry feelings.

Rebecca doesn't expect a great change in Sam's behaviour. Sam is young and doesn't have the physical and emotional maturity to deal with his turbulent feelings consistently, although he may well become more skilled at controlling his moods and expressing them in different ways. The best Rebecca can do is show support and not make Sam feel that he is being rejected because of his moods and tantrums. She keeps the channels of communication open and uses her skills in communication and listening to tune in to Sam's feelings and make it as easy as she can for him to speak about them. Rebecca uses phrases like:

'That really got to you, didn't it.'
'You sound really angry and upset.'
'That's tough.'

She tries to be ready to talk when Sam wants to, and to be alert for opportunities to discover what he is thinking and feeling.

Tips for handling teenage anger

- Don't give up on the situation, or the child.
- Don't take it personally – even if the attack seems to be aimed at you, the feelings behind it are likely to be more complex.
- Make it easy for them to back off without losing face.
- Don't put them down.
- Don't say that you know how they feel – use reflection. Instead of 'I know how you feel' try 'It sounds as if you are angry because of what happened at break time.'
- Don't make comparisons with what you were like at that age.
- Don't preach or play the 'I'm the one in charge' card.
- Do stick to the boundaries that have been established.
- Be ready to negotiate boundaries as circumstances change.
- Present a good role model – how you manage your anger will send a message.
- Keep your sense of humour – but be careful not to let them think that you are laughing at them or not taking them seriously.
- If there are two of you in the parenting role, agree on a consistent approach.
- Encourage a problem-solving approach – don't take over or jump in with solutions.
- Be aware – uncontrollable or unfathomable moods may be signs of depression.

Premenstrual moods

Your oestrogen and progesterone levels vary throughout the month, and when your oestrogen levels fall, in the middle of your monthly cycle, you may feel tense and irritable, and be liable to fly off the handle or burst into tears at the slightest thing.

If you know that your irritability occurs when you are premenstrual, there might be some steps that you can take to lessen the degree to which you become tetchy. Identify the things that get you particularly annoyed at this time – it might be the house being in a mess, or the children being difficult, or feeling that you don't have enough support. Once you are aware of the times when you get snappy or aggressive you can prepare to deal with these occasions by using thought-calming techniques and physical relaxation. Remember that you can't help the feelings that are stimulated, but you can choose how you deal with them. You may choose to run with the snappiness, knowing that it won't last for ever, or you may choose to deal with the situation to minimize the discomfort for you and for others.

There may be some practical things you can do to help you feel more in control. This might be a good time to arrange for some help if it is appropriate and available, or to arrange for some time to yourself if that is what you need. You could keep an eye on the calendar and make sure that you don't over-commit yourself in the days when you may feel stressed and uptight.

Baby blues

The physical and emotional upheaval of giving birth can trigger a range of difficult feelings. Even an easy birth and a wonderful baby can cause stress and anxiety as lack of sleep and constantly being in demand take their toll and cause you to be moody, tearful and irritable. If these feelings don't go away, and if you have bouts of anger and rage, maybe directed at your partner or your family, or at your baby, or at yourself, don't keep your state of mind to yourself. Anger can be one of the signs of postnatal depression, so don't struggle on hoping that things will improve. Talk to your doctor or health care worker. There are voluntary organizations and support networks which can offer you practical and emotional help.

Menopausal swings

Fluctuating hormone levels at this stage of life may cause you to have the kind of mood swings you experienced when you were younger, and you may find that your anger is triggered frequently and unexpectedly.

You can maintain some control over your emotional state by recognizing and accepting that your mood is temporary and won't last.

Talk about what's going on with you

You may like to acknowledge the cyclical nature of your moods. It might be helpful to explain to particular individuals in your life that you know you are irritable at these times. Plan carefully how you are going to communicate this, and be sure not to apologize or blame yourself for physical changes in your body, or for legitimate anger.

Don't let your feelings be dismissed

Don't be too ready to dismiss your irritability as occurring solely because it's that time of the month. You may have genuine grievances which make you healthily angry which come out when you are feeling vulnerable and which you suppress the rest of the time. If this is the case, then think about how to address these issues. At the same time, don't allow others to write off your behaviour as being purely hormone-driven.

Loss and bereavement

In the period following loss or bereavement you are likely to be angry with a range of people. You may rail against doctors, solicitors, the health service, the legal system. You are even more likely to be angry and confrontational with those close to you. In your distress and helplessness, and your sense of how unfair the world is, you need to find someone to blame, and you hit out at anyone near you. This is part of the grieving process. If you find that it goes on for a long time and if your anger becomes very unmanageable, you might need to see your doctor or a counsellor about getting some help.

Lifting your mood

As we have seen, it is important to recognize and explore our negative moods, and take note of what they tell us. Then, it is helpful not to wallow in or indulge feelings of anger, misery or frustration, but to try to lift yourself to a higher, more buoyant frame of mind. Try to do something which will boost your energy levels and raise you out of that draggy, just-below-par condition that is familiar to us all at some time or other, and that can lead to tetchy and angry behaviour.

Some of the following suggestions will work for you. Strategies which involve you taking an active role may be the most effective in the long run. Experiment until you have found a good way of altering your mood for the better.

Use your body

If your body behaves in an upbeat way, your mind and your mood will rise to the occasion:

- Smile. Even if you don't feel like smiling inside, the action produces some helpful hormones that make you feel better.
- Laugh. Laughter is an even more potent way of releasing endorphins into your body.
- Walk tall. Make your posture upright and relaxed, being sure not to tense any muscles as you do so. Move and walk in the way that upbeat, confident people do. Take purposeful steps, keep your head up. This physical lift will lift you internally as well.
- Do something physical. Energetic physical activity is a great mood-lifter. Find an activity you enjoy doing and that you can do easily without having to make arrangements and preparations. Walking or jogging fits the bill very well, and there is added benefit if you can do this in a place where there is some natural colour and greenery.
- If you enjoy activities such as cooking or decorating, this would be a good time to engage in them. Baking a cake, making a delicious recipe, transforming a room will have a positive effect on your mood. So will doing some clearing or de-cluttering – just a little bit of time spent clearing a cupboard or tidying a drawer will have practical and psychological benefits, smoothing the rough edges of your environment and creating a feeling of calm.

Use your mind

Find a strategy or two that helps your mind to focus on things that make you feel more upbeat:

- Identify three things that are good about your life. Write them down.
- Identify three things that you have done well recently.
- Make a mental or written store of incidents and memories that always make you smile or feel warm. Choose one of them and relive that moment.
- Rather than think about and dwell on your low feelings, use the kind of reframing and positive self-talk which we discussed earlier.
- Do something that makes you feel that you can control and influence parts of your life – plan a holiday, make a list of things to do this week, tidy a cupboard.
- Listen to music. Music can relax or elevate your mood. Experiment until you find the kind of music that helps you feel the way you want to.

Social activity

Engaging with other people works on several different levels:

- Have a chat with a friend about what has been bothering you.
- Have a chat with a friend about different matters entirely.
- Do something to help someone else – volunteer your time, or a skill or service you can offer.
- Drag yourself out to the party or the PTA social or the hen night even if you don't feel like it – making the effort and having to talk to people mobilizes energy and lifts your mood.

Give yourself a treat

Pampering and the rituals of self-care can help to make you feel better:

- Take a long relaxing bath.
- Prepare something nice to eat.
- Buy yourself something fun and affordable – a new lipstick works for many women.

- Have a beauty treatment such as a facial or manicure.
- Get your hair done.
- Start a novel you have been saving up to read.
- Go to an exhibition.
- Eat something delicious.

Chill out

Engaging in passive activities can help:

- Watch something undemanding on TV.
- Rent a feel-good DVD.
- Read a distracting magazine.
- Have a short nap.
- Sit quietly with a soothing drink.

Unreliable mood-lifters

Stimulants

Drinking stimulants such as caffeine, eating something sugary, having a glass of wine or a cigarette can give us an immediate boost. The effect is only temporary, though, and these activities can't be relied on for long-term mood management.

Anger and alcohol

The immediate effect of a glass of wine probably is to make you feel relaxed. It takes away some of your stress and anxiety and helps you to wind down. However, alcohol is essentially a depressant of the central nervous system. Its effect is to trigger angry feelings – we all know people who get punchy and aggressive after they've had a few drinks – and it affects your ability to communicate and think clearly. If you get on the attack when you've been drinking, think about the nature of the feelings that rise to the surface, and acknowledge what those hidden emotions are telling you.

Getting rid of unexpected and unwanted anger

Sometimes a flare-up of anger can take us by surprise. You think that you are in control of a situation and that you are not experiencing any hostile thoughts or reactions, then suddenly something flicks on the raw – something someone says or does, or something you see or hear or read, pushes the button and you feel your body leaping into fighting mode.

What you need to do immediately is to calm your body down and get rid of your physical tension. It is helpful if you learn to recognize your own particular warning signs of an imminent explosion. You might be aware of your heart beating more quickly and your breathing speeding up. Your stomach might start fluttering or churning, and you may feel waves of panic. You might go very hot or very cold, very twitchy or very still, as if you have been immobilized. Perhaps your hands go into fists, or your jaw becomes tense and rigid. As soon as you recognize what is happening, act quickly to counteract the stress response. The following processes take place simultaneously.

Physical relaxation

Consciously relax your muscles. Start with the areas of your body which have gone into 'fight' mode – unclench your fists, drop your shoulders, loosen your jaw, unclench your toes. Let your arms and hands relax. You will feel your tension begin to drain away. If you are with another person or people, you may need to remove yourself for a few moments.

Calm breathing

When our anger is triggered we start to breathe quickly from high up in the chest, and our tension level rises. To counteract this effect, take a deep breath starting from way down in your diaphragm. Count to five as you draw in breath through your nose. Feel your chest rise. Breathe out slowly and completely, expelling all the air that you have taken in. Keep your chest still, and feel your stomach muscles rise and fall. Do this once or twice.

As you breathe in, you could say to yourself, 'Calm in'; and as you breathe out you could think, 'Tension out'. Find words that work for you.

Manage your thoughts

When your body is calm you are more able to apply thought processes to the situation. However you want to deal with it, you will be effective only if you are in control of your reaction and responding from a state of calmness. Use some steadying self-talk:

'Hang on now.'
'This is something I can cope with.'
'I won't let this overwhelm me.'
'I can stay cool.'

Get rid of angry thoughts

Treat these unbidden angry intrusions as irritating pests that you can swat away. Imagine yourself batting them into oblivion.

Just focus on the word 'Stop!' Imagine the word written in large letters, dancing in front of your eyes like a pop-up on a computer screen. Hear the word in your head. Hear yourself shouting the word as loudly as you can. If you are alone, you could actually shout it out.

Think blue. Get rid of red rage by bathing the whole scene in icy cool blue.

Distract yourself

Stay calm by focusing your mind on something neutral. Choose an object in the room and describe it to yourself.

Recite to yourself something you don't have to think about – the days of the week, the months of the year. Recite them backwards.

Choose an object in your vision and concentrate on it – it might be a piece of furniture, a cup, a curtain. Study it as if you are going to have to give a detailed description of it in a few minutes' time.

Count backwards from ten.

Laugh it away

Humour is a powerful tool in the fight against anger. Bring yourself out of your angry state by turning your reactions into funny, exaggerated images – see yourself as a baby throwing a rattle out of a pram, or imagine yourself jumping up and down and squeaking.

Remember, you are not laughing at yourself for feeling angry. What you are doing is finding a way of lifting your tense and hostile mood. You can examine the nature and cause of your angry mood later, if that is what you need to do.

How to stop your anger taking hold

If you act quickly enough when you recognize the first signs of anger you may be able to become calm enough to manage the mood before it develops. There is a range of different early-warning signals to watch out for. Get to know your own particular behavioural signs, the indications that tell you that you may be building up to an angry outbreak.

These indications will vary from person to person. Apart from the physical signs of the stress response, some of us have our own little behavioural habits which indicate that there is a storm brewing. Amy notices that she starts to tap on the table. Karen starts to hum under her breath. Louise suddenly feels that she can't sit still, and walks around aimlessly.

Exercise 8.2: Warning signals

What are the signals that warn you that you are getting agitated? (You may not be aware of these, so you could ask someone who knows you well to help you identify signs.)

Things I do

_____

_____

_____

Things I say

_____

_____

_____

9

Handling anger in public

Rage on the roads

Physical assaults caused by road rage are the most extreme manifestations of the anger and frustration that are often experienced by road users. Less dramatic than out-and-out assaults, but still dangerous to our physical and mental well-being, are the kinds of verbal and non-verbal threats and aggressive responses that all too frequently occur. Some drivers become furious when other road users drive in a way that they consider to be inappropriate – going too fast or too slow, tailgating, overtaking, cutting in, being in the wrong lane or, as they see it, simply driving like idiots. Even people who are generally calm can become stressed and angry when they encounter drivers they perceive as in some way breaking the written and unwritten rules of sharing road space. Sometimes our anger is ignited because our safety is threatened by someone's dangerous driving; sometimes we become angry when our self-esteem and sense of personal worth are undermined by a driver's behaviour; sometimes we become enraged because our plans are being thwarted and we are held up or otherwise inconvenienced by travel conditions. It is almost as if being in a car can make us ultra-sensitive to the presence of potential threats and assaults, and heightens our need for self-protection and our desire to get what we want and have life be the way we want it to be. Although rationally we know that we cannot count on any journey to be trouble-free and without any unexpected or unwelcome elements, we react fiercely and violently to disruptions and obstacles, whether they are caused by other people or by external events.

Exercise 9.1: Road rage

Do you suffer from road rage? Mark the following situations on a scale of 1 to 10, 1 indicating that the situation doesn't bother you and 10 indicating that the situation really makes you mad.

Anyone driving too fast	1 2 3 4 5 6 7 8 9 10
Younger people driving too fast	1 2 3 4 5 6 7 8 9 10
Older people driving too fast	1 2 3 4 5 6 7 8 9 10
Anyone driving too slowly	1 2 3 4 5 6 7 8 9 10
Younger people driving too slowly	1 2 3 4 5 6 7 8 9 10
Older people driving too slowly	1 2 3 4 5 6 7 8 9 10
Someone cutting in too close	1 2 3 4 5 6 7 8 9 10
Erratic lane-changing	1 2 3 4 5 6 7 8 9 10
Tailgating	1 2 3 4 5 6 7 8 9 10
Ignoring traffic signals	1 2 3 4 5 6 7 8 9 10
Poor or late signalling	1 2 3 4 5 6 7 8 9 10
Being stuck in a queue or traffic jam	1 2 3 4 5 6 7 8 9 10
Someone pulling out without looking	1 2 3 4 5 6 7 8 9 10
Driving on full beam	1 2 3 4 5 6 7 8 9 10
4 x 4s being driven in town	1 2 3 4 5 6 7 8 9 10
Children being driven to school in 4 x 4s	1 2 3 4 5 6 7 8 9 10
Cigarette butts being thrown out of car windows	1 2 3 4 5 6 7 8 9 10
Rubbish being thrown out of car windows	1 2 3 4 5 6 7 8 9 10
Drivers talking on mobile phones	1 2 3 4 5 6 7 8 9 10
Drivers turning round to talk to children in the back	1 2 3 4 5 6 7 8 9 10
Loud music on car radios	1 2 3 4 5 6 7 8 9 10
Parking in disabled bays	1 2 3 4 5 6 7 8 9 10
Parking in parent-and-child bays	1 2 3 4 5 6 7 8 9 10
Taking up two parking spaces	1 2 3 4 5 6 7 8 9 10
Taking the parking space you had your eye on	1 2 3 4 5 6 7 8 9 10
Anyone driving the model of car you would like but can't afford	1 2 3 4 5 6 7 8 9 10

Add your own ideas:

_____

_____

_____

Beliefs about other people which can lead to road rage

Our anger when on the road is not incited directly by other people's driving and behaviour, but by the way that this challenges our beliefs and ideas about the way that people should behave behind the wheel of a car. Depending on how strongly you hold these beliefs, your anger is triggered when you are confronted by ways of driving which violate them. As you register that this violation is taking place you are fired with indignation, which can quickly erupt into intense anger. What you can do to prevent the leap to an angry response is change the way that you think about these trigger situations.

Some of the ideas about other people which are challenged by the driving behaviour of others include:

- People should drive considerately.
- No one has the right to put another's well-being in danger.
- People should not be allowed to drive in that way.
- People should show more responsibility.
- People should respect each other.
- The roads should be kept in better condition.
- Something should be done about this kind of driver.

Add your own ideas:

_____

_____

_____

Beliefs about ourselves which can lead to road rage

Our thoughts about ourselves and what we are entitled to can lead to furious reactions when it seems to us that we are not getting what we deserve. Some of these ideas include:

- Anyone who behaves badly to me is showing disrespect.
- I have the right to get where I am going within the time frame that I choose.
- I have the right not be inconvenienced.

- I have the right to fair treatment at all times.
- I need to be in control all the time.

Add your own ideas:

_____

_____

_____

Faulty assumptions and interpretations which can lead to road rage

Consciously or subconsciously we make judgements about people's motives and thoughts. Here are some typical assumptions:

- Others make things difficult for me on purpose.
- That was deliberate.
- That person was obviously out to get me.
- People driving bigger cars than mine think they are superior to me.
- Those people don't care about how their driving affects me and others.
- They obviously think they're above the law.

Add your own ideas:

_____

_____

_____

How to calm road rage by changing your beliefs

Instead of winding yourself up thinking how people should behave, lower your stress level by accepting that although you would like people to behave in a certain way, they don't have to, and perhaps they don't know how to in any case.

Accept that you cannot make other people better drivers. What you can do is be a considerate driver yourself.

Accept that you cannot stop others from wanting to get ahead, to grab what they want. What you can do is refuse to be influenced by their emotional state and their needs.

How to calm road rage by broadening your way of interpreting events

Give people the benefit of the doubt – when you don't know for certain that something is done on purpose, decide that it is not deliberate, but a mistake. Remind yourself that you cannot read others' thoughts and you cannot assume that your interpretation of their motives is accurate.

Accept that other drivers may be tired, upset, hungry, anxious.

Accept that some people, whether they realize it or not, are poor drivers with a low level of competence behind the wheel.

Accept that attacks or affronts are not personal. The other driver does not know you and is not out to get you. He or she is feeling frustrated and thwarted.

Feel sorry for dangerous or erratic drivers – they are far more likely to come to grief than skilful and careful drivers like you.

When you get wound up, don't claim immediate 100 per cent rage. Tell yourself: 'That was a bit irritating', 'That was a trifle out of order.'

Exercise 9.2: Looking at things differently

Imagine that:

You are driving slowly along a narrow country lane, looking for the turn-off that you need. Suddenly a car comes right up behind you and beeps for you to get out of the way. You are forced to veer to the left and you overshoot your turning as the car behind overtakes you.

Which of the following reflects your thoughts and feelings?

- They shouldn't be allowed on the road.
- I hope they have an accident.
- People who drive so aggressively should have their licence taken away for good.

Add your own ideas:

_____

_____

_____

Imagine that:

The other driver in the above scene was driving in that way because:

- He was rushing to hospital with his wife who had suddenly gone into labour.
- She was rushing to hospital with her child who was having breathing difficulties.

How have your thoughts and feelings changed?

Of course, a dangerous or frustrating situation remains so whatever the circumstances – but you will get less angry and worked up if you change the way that you think about the incident.

Ways to stay calm and minimize anger on the road

- Choose whatever you listen to in your car with care – certain types of music or talk programme can keep you calm, while others may have the opposite effect.
- Allow as much time as you can for your journey.
- Accept that you may be delayed.
- Decide how you will deal with potential hold-ups.
- Drive as considerately as you can. Act the role of the courteous and non-combative driver – let people go in front of you, smile if they cut in. After all, their need is obviously greater than yours.
- Mentally run a third-person commentary on your driving: 'Now she will very calmly indicate and pull out. She knows she is driving safely.' (The use of the third person, 'she', helps you to remain detached and unemotional.)
- Keep your body relaxed – don't grip the steering wheel or tense your shoulders.
- If you are the perceived aggressor, don't get drawn into an argument. Keep your doors and windows shut.
- Always make an apologetic sign, even if you think you are not in the wrong.
- In confrontational situations, don't make eye contact with other drivers.
- Always thank other drivers.
- On a long journey, don't put off taking a break.
- Don't invest too much of your identity in your vehicle. You may love it and it may be essential to your life, but it is only a metal contraption. It is not worth more than your mental well-being. It is not worth dying for.

Rage in the air

Air travel is stressful. We are at the mercy of crowds, of huge delays, of cancellations. Increased security checks take longer and are more demanding. We are surrounded by strangers, some of whom may be drinking too much, some of whom may be loud and aggressive. This category may include family members and travelling companions. We are hurtling through the clouds miles above the earth, confined in an unnaturally small space, breathing recycled air. We may be tired, hungry and thirsty. With these continual assaults on our physical and mental comfort, our anger can be easily triggered, leading in extreme cases to the situations which hit the headlines. Maybe the most remarkable thing is not that there are so many air rage incidents, but that there aren't even more.

Decide to be calm

Travelling by air means relinquishing control, a circumstance which can unbalance us and heighten our anxiety levels. Although we have no control over the external aspects of our journey, we can take responsibility for our thoughts and attitudes. Make a decision before you travel that you will not allow yourself to get angry and worked up about the frustrations that you will probably encounter.

Choose a calming phrase to use when you begin to get tense and angry:

'I'm not going to let this get to me.'
'This will be over soon.'
'This is only a journey from a to b, it is not a major life event.'

Anticipate problems

Whether your flight is for pleasure or for business, part of your planning is based on the assumption that the journey will go smoothly. While you don't want to approach your holiday or your meeting in a negative frame of mind, you are more likely to keep calm in the face of disruptions if you build in an expectation that things might not go exactly according to plan. Deciding in advance how you will deal with these circumstances helps you to feel in control, and it could mean that you respond more with resignation than with anger when the plane is delayed, or you want to get to sleep and can't, or you don't like any of the films being shown.

Exercise 9.3: What triggers your anger?

Identify the situations which are likely to trigger your anger. They might include:

Delays and cancellations
Luggage being lost or mislaid
Other people's behaviour
Family members/children being annoying
Not liking your seat
Being physically uncomfortable
Being tired
Feeling bored
Unexpected occurrences

Add your own ideas:

_____

_____

_____

Decide how you will deal with problems

Think about how you will remain calm if these situations occur. Write down what you will think, what you will do, and visualize yourself coping with the circumstance.

Exercise 9.4: How will you keep calm?

Choose the three situations which are most likely to get you tense and worked up. Decide what you will do to keep calm if this situation arises.

Situation	What I will think	What I will do
1		
2		
3		

Do some practical preparation

You can lessen the effect of some of these situations by taking some practical steps to increase your comfort and well-being.

Find out exactly what weight and type of luggage you can take.
Pack basic essentials in your hand luggage.

Find out what security checks are in place.

Make a checklist of necessary airport items and tick them off as they are put in the appropriate place.

Plan your journey to the airport. Don't make an automatic assumption that there is only one way of getting there, or that what you usually do will be best. Explore all modes of available transport and parking options, taking into account your time of travel, any individual needs that should be catered for, etc. (You could apply a problem-solving approach to this and other decisions.)

Gauge the optimum time of arrival at the airport. You don't want the stress of feeling rushed and anxious about missing the plane, nor do you want the stress of hanging around for too long.

Choose what you need for distraction and entertainment. It may be that your usual choices and resources in reading matter, music, DVDs, games won't work for you in quite the same way when travelling as they do at home, or they might be just what you need. Make your decision carefully – you can feel surprisingly edgy if you find on the plane that you've already read the book that you planned would occupy you for most of the flight, or that the comedy all your friends raved about isn't amusing you, or the Sudoku or word puzzles you've taken with you are too easy or too difficult.

Nervous flyers

Fear may cause you to be jumpy and wound up. There are many books, programmes and resources available to help people overcome their fears and stay calm. You could think about investing some time in tracking down something that might work for you.

Travelling with babies and children

Feeling anxious about the well-being and behaviour of young family members is likely to put you on edge, and there is always the possibility that their behaviour will irritate other passengers. Don't leave things to chance and hope for the best – check out the wealth of suggestions available in books and online about how to make flying with children as temper-free as possible. You will find recommendations about child-friendly (and not-so-friendly) airlines, about the kind of practical support that is available on board, about ways of helping restless kids to be settled, and a host of good ideas based on other people's experiences.

Staying calm on public transport

Even short journeys on buses or trains can cause annoyance and anger. Discomfort, noise, overcrowding and inconsiderate behaviour are among the irritants which can result in you arriving at your destination in a snappy mood. You can insulate yourself from the potentially damaging effects of fraught journeys by applying the same thought processes and practical suggestions as we discussed above with reference to air travel.

Peace train

Naomi finds her train commute to work very stressful. Her nerves are on edge as she has to endure inevitable delays, loud conversations on mobile phones, irritating habits of fellow passengers. She gets worked up as she imagines just what she would like to say or do to that person who is inflicting details of his day's schedule on everyone within earshot, and she has to restrain herself from viciously elbowing anyone who brushes against her as they get on or off the train. If she tries to read or work on her laptop she can't concentrate. Naomi jokes that one day she will do something that will get her arrested, but it actually isn't funny.

Amanda travels the same route. She physically cuts out distracting noise by listening to music that she likes and makes her feel good, or she uses ear plugs. On the occasions when she cannot avoid hearing annoying conversations, she amuses herself by making up stories about the person speaking. Another strategy she uses if she finds her annoyance levels rising is to reframe the situation. Instead of thinking how infuriating someone is being, she thinks:

'That person has hearing problems and doesn't realize how loudly he is speaking.'
'That person who bumped into me is distracted because she had bad news this morning.'

When her train is delayed or doesn't turn up, she tells herself that she can't do anything about it, so she can use the time to do something specific: read a newspaper, read another chapter of her book, plan a new wardrobe, go over stuff for work . . .

She chooses to travel in the designated 'quiet carriage' whenever possible.

Shops, pavements, people ...

Our leisure activities and daily routines can be turned into mini-assault courses by the number of irritating factors that need to be overcome before we can buy what we need or even make our way to the shop or cinema or café. You might feel like snapping at or pushing aside people who walk too slowly, or who stay in groups taking up the whole pavement, or who don't seem to recognize the concept of queuing, not to mention those who suddenly stop walking to speak on their mobile phones. Shopping with children or partners in tow can turn the high street into a battleground. You can manage these occasions more effectively by identifying the situations which really get to you, and preparing to deal with them.

Manage your expectations

The first step to remaining calm in these circumstances is not to expect your outing to be trouble-free. Thinking 'It will only take me a few minutes to pick up these items' or 'I'll just nip along to the Monsoon sale at lunchtime' or 'We'll all have a nice time shopping then go for a family meal' is a potential recipe for frustration and bad temper. Always assume that something will take longer than you think and allow extra time. Always bear in mind that others on your expedition will have their own needs and agendas, and are likely to be difficult if these are not met.

Manage the crowds

If you can't stand people getting in your way as you try to get from a to b, decide on some strategies which will stop you getting worked up.

Play the part of being a cheery pavement user. Smile and say a pleasant but firm 'Excuse me' when you want to pass someone. Decide to forgive people who have poor pavement manners. Tell yourself that it isn't their fault that they don't know how to behave.

Read the street. A little bit of observation can smooth your way to a more trouble-free passage. It may be that everyone is entering a shop through a busy main entrance, but there might be a side or back entrance which is far less used. It may take a few more minutes to get to it, but it could be worth it to avoid the crowds. You may be able to avoid pavement crowds by cutting through a shop.

Ask yourself if you really want to waste valuable anger on this crowd of strangers. You can use your anger energy in far more productive ways.

Manage the shops

Being stuck in a queue with only one or two tills operating can be infuriating. Tapping your foot impatiently and constantly looking at your watch just reminds you that you're angry. Decide whether you want to address the situation or not. If you don't want to take any action, then stay calm by switching off and turning your mind to something else, or reframe the circumstances by thinking, 'Here's a chance to pause and stop rushing.' If you want to do something about the situation, the best thing is to catch the attention of an assistant, either one serving or one passing, and say something like: 'We've been waiting a long time here. Could you open another till or do something to sort it out?'

Poor service can get you riled. You will feel calm and in control if you express your displeasure without losing your temper. If an individual is giving you bad service, decide precisely what is poor about it. Is it lack of attention, not listening to what you are asking, carrying on another conversation at the same time? Calmly and firmly, state what you would like to happen: 'I'd appreciate your help now'; 'I can see you're talking to your colleague, but I would like to be attended to.' If, on the other hand, an over-attentive assistant's hovering is getting to you, say, with a smile, something like: 'I'd prefer to look round on my own, thanks.'

When you receive good service, try telling the person that you appreciate it. Not just a routine thank-you – say something like 'You have been very patient. I really appreciate that' or 'Thank you for taking the time to search that out.' Your comment will be appreciated and will lift the mood of the person who receives it, you will feel good for having expressed pleasure, and you will have created a tiny drop of well-being in a tetchy environment.

It may not surprise you to hear that tempers are most frequently lost in the shops on busy Saturday afternoons. So be prepared to exercise your anger management strategies if you must shop at this time – or make other arrangements so that you avoid this flash-point time.

In the workplace

There may be many causes for justified, healthy anger at work. Apart from the tensions and frustrations that everyone experiences, there can be additional pressure on women in the workplace. Many women are trying to meet the demands of their home life and their work life, as well as shouldering major responsibilities for child care and household chores, or care for elderly parents or relatives. There are issues about inequality of pay and opportunities for promotion. Women may experience barriers or resentment from colleagues about flexible working hours, and in workplaces where there is a child-oriented or family-friendly approach to taking time off, making use of it too frequently, in others' eyes, can cause problems with co-workers.

Helen loses it

Helen has returned to work after maternity leave, taking up her old position as team leader. She does her job well, but she finds that she has to put twice as much energy into achieving the same level of results as before. She feels tired, and as the day goes on she becomes anxious about leaving in time to pick Lily up from the childminder. She feels that Jason, who did her job in her absence, is just waiting for her to slip up, and this makes her tense and self-conscious. One day she mislabels a sample in the laboratory, and Jason makes some crack about her having lost her touch. This flicks Helen on the raw, and she finds herself yelling at Jason to get off her case. Their boss hears what's going on, and calls Helen in for a discussion about how she's coping.

Helen let her feelings build up until she had this explosion of anger. During the build-up period she didn't think rationally about her situation, because she was too occupied with just surviving. When she addresses it as a problem, and doesn't just put her feelings down to stress and tiredness, she can identify one of the aspects as Jason's attitude to her. Dealing with this calmly and assertively will help Helen keep her feelings in perspective and put their working relationship on to a different footing. However, she now also has to deal with her boss's perception of her as someone who's not managing things very well.

Gender divide

No matter what the provocation, it is not a good idea for women or men to lose their tempers or behave aggressively or have a tantrum at work. The unfortunate case is that when a man behaves like this, he can get away with it. Such behaviour is sometimes, of course mistakenly, seen as a badge of power or authority. An angry woman, on the other hand, is seen as out of control, or as a bitch, depending on her level of seniority.

Men gain respect from some people when they behave in this way, whereas women lose respect and status, and their competency is drawn into question.

Tears at work

Many of us will have experienced feeling so angry and worked up about something that we find ourselves bursting into tears. Again, this response is likely to be perceived in a negative way by those who interpret such a reaction as an indication of weakness and lack of control, the mark of someone who can't take criticism or is incompetent or who cannot handle difficult situations.

Managing your feelings

In the public arena of the workplace, it will probably be to your advantage to express your anger in a controlled and assertive way. When you feel that you're about to snap at someone, or when the tears start in your eyes, you need to regain a sense of calm. Take a couple of deep breaths and practise whatever self-calming strategies work for you. (Look at the suggestions on pp. 101–2.) It's not too late to do this even if you've already shown anger by shouting or bursting into tears. As soon as you can, say something like, 'As you can see, this has really got to me. I'm going to take five minutes', and remove yourself from the situation.

Once you are calm you will be able to apply rational thought to probe your feelings and identify the core of your anger. Then you can decide if you need to do something about it, and think about who you need to speak to. When you are ready, have the appropriate conversation with the appropriate person.

Making the most of your emotional responses

Your anger at work, as in any situation, is a sign that something is wrong. Don't feel ashamed of responding emotionally – being emotionally aware is a great asset in every area of life. Use this awareness to develop your skills of observation, empathy and communication, so that these become the distinguishing features of your working style.

10

How to live more peacefully

As well as managing anger positively and constructively, look for ways of not getting angry in the first place. This is not to suggest that you should lose the fire that energizes you to deal with things that are wrong, or that you should just become accepting of damage and hurt – that is not the path to a healthy existence. But you could think about cultivating a way of life and a way of being that embraces peace and calmness rather than shutting it out.

Getting rid of anger

When you get angry, how long does the feeling last? When you have experienced that powerful surge of emotion, what happens to it? What should happen is that after not too long your anger subsides. Of course, this is not to say that you then forget about the problem, but that you let go of the feelings that have engulfed you, and allow your mind and body to return to a state of calm. If you allow anger to hang on, and if you actually encourage it by going over and over the same ground in your thoughts, you are likely to damage yourself physically and emotionally. It may not surprise you to hear that women tend to hang on to their anger for longer than men, often bottling it up until one day it explodes. Wanting not to be angry is a stepping stone to a more peaceful existence.

Unresolved issues

Sometimes our anger is not really to do with what's going on now, but is to do with things that happened in the past. Perhaps you use your anger or hang on to angry feelings as a way of protecting yourself from other emotions. There may be psychological and emotional wounds from your childhood, of which you may be unaware, colouring the way that you experience anger now. You may have had painful experiences of abuse or injustice or

119

loss which remain under the surface of your skin and emerge in unexpected and powerful ways when you are under pressure or in situations that consciously or subconsciously recall the past.

A shadow from the past

Joan finds herself quite irrationally scared of her new boss. Louise has rather a brusque manner, and has been heard to say that she doesn't suffer fools gladly. Joan's feelings are getting in the way of her performance at work – she speaks to Louise as little as possible, and makes excuses for putting off meetings.

Joan realizes that Louise reminds her of her old gym teacher, a bullying woman who used to mock Joan for her timidity and ineptitude at games. Joan used to feel intimidated and thought that she was useless and incompetent. With the help of a supportive friend, Joan thinks it through and acknowledges that there is loads of evidence from her life to prove that she is not useless and incompetent. She can leave those feelings in the past where they belong and channel her energies into building a good relationship with Louise and proving her worth as a team member. Although Louise has something of an intimidating manner, Joan can now relate to her without being influenced by her old experience.

If you find that your reaction to a person or situation is out of proportion to the circumstances, it could be something from the past that is troubling you. You may be over-reacting to your perception of threat because of the aggressive behaviour you received before. Before you can address the present situation, you need to examine these left-over feelings and separate them from what is going on now.

Healing and forgiveness

There is a body of opinion that says you cannot heal the past until you have forgiven those who harmed you. Others acknowledge that some hurts cannot be forgiven, and that what you need to do is find a way of moving on even though you are unable to forgive what was done to you. It is important that you do move on and let go of your anger, or else you are suffering over and over again for something which has happened, is over, and which you have no power to change.

Forgiving isn't easy. It's particularly hard when the person who hurt you will not or cannot show remorse, and you may need to get rid of your desire or expectation to hear these words. What you might try is beginning by forgiving people for smaller offences – your first boyfriend for dumping you, your old teacher for saying you would never amount to anything, your parents for moving house so that you were miles away from your friends ... These may seem trivial events, but this kind of occurrence can cause us to get angry and worked up, even years later, particularly if we are looking for ways of fanning the flame of anger by quoting examples of wrongs that were done to us way back in the past.

If there are major experiences in your life that you want to forgive but find it difficult to do so, find help from expert support. Although you can learn to leave anger behind and live in a peaceful way, forgiveness has huge emotional and spiritual benefits.

Living with triggers you cannot escape

Of course, emotional reactions can be triggered suddenly and unexpectedly, but it is likely that there is a pattern in the way that you respond to particular people and events. Get to know the kinds of situations which are likely to spark an angry reaction in you. Some of these situations will be constant presences in your life – family members and work colleagues who are part of your daily life, friendships you want to continue but which have provoking elements, and other irritants which get under your skin. Have a strategy ready to help you deal with the situation.

Exercise 10.1: Who gets under your skin?

Use the suggestions in Chapter 3 to help you to identify precisely the people and situations which require you to manage your feelings consciously in order to prevent yourself getting wound up and annoyed.

Jot down the names of the people whose language or behaviour is predictable and which always gets to you. Decide how you will deal with it in the future.

Person: *My sister-in-law*
What they do/say: *'That little bit of extra weight suits you.'*
How I usually respond: *Flare of anger. Grit teeth and smile. Feel put down.*
How I will deal with it from now on: *Check angry response. Tell myself I am not going to let her make me feel bad. Say: 'Thanks. I'm pleased with the way I look at the moment.'*

Person _____

What they do/say _____

How I usually respond _____

How I will deal with it from now on _____

Person _____

What they do/say _____

How I usually respond _____

How I will deal with it from now on _____

Person _____

What they do/say _____

How I usually respond _____

How I will deal with it from now on _____

Focusing on your long-term emotional well-being

Increasing self-esteem

People with high self-esteem are good at managing anger. Having a good level of self-esteem doesn't mean that you think too much of yourself, or that you are smug or self-satisfied. It means that you know and accept yourself, that you acknowledge your faults and weaknesses without letting them colour and diminish your worth as a person. Because your sense of your own identity is sound, you have nothing to prove. You are aware of your own needs and know how to manage situations in which they are not being met without playing games or becoming inappropriately angry.

Physical exercise

Regular exercise helps to keep your spirits up as well as improving your physical well-being. It increases your energy levels, lowers your blood pressure and strengthens your immune system. Don't leave it until you feel an angry mood coming on and want to work it off – try to make moderate exercise a part of your everyday life. Aerobic exercise is among the most beneficial. The vigorous movement involved in walking briskly, jogging or running, dancing and playing certain sports makes your heart pump efficiently and allows you to discharge your energy. Exercise also releases mood-elevating endorphins into your bloodstream; these, and the boost of adrenalin you get immediately after exercising, create a feel-good factor which is great for your emotional health.

If going to a gym or something similar wouldn't work for you, find ways of incorporating physical activity into your everyday life so that you don't have to make a big deal of it. You could choose to walk short distances rather than drive – 20 minutes' brisk walking is the beneficial level. Go up and down stairs rather than using lifts. Put on upbeat music at home and dance or move around as you do household chores.

Add your own ideas:

_____

_____

_____

Schedule time for yourself

Looking after yourself and seeing to your own needs is not an additional extra, a kind of bolt-on that you attend to if there's time. For many women the pressures of being constantly on call for others and being constantly aware of others' needs can give rise to anger and resentment. Make a point of nurturing yourself as well as everyone else. Do something which you enjoy, which nourishes your sense of yourself and replenishes your resources. Only you know what these activities are. Make a note of them in Exercise 10.2.

Exercise 10.2: Nurturing yourself

What I could do with ten minutes _____

_____

What I could do with half an hour _____

_____

What I could do with a morning or afternoon _____

_____

What I could do with a day _____

_____

Cultivating optimism

Healthy optimism is different from unrealistic thinking about the future. A balanced, optimistic outlook is one which looks for the good in situations and does not look for or focus on the negative. Such an outlook gives you a robust attitude to life, and its benefits include the fact that optimism helps you deal with disappointment and frustration in a positive way and protects you from slipping into the negative frames of mind which are linked with anger and depression. This doesn't mean to say that you shut your eyes to bad things that happen, only that you do not allow them to overwhelm you. An optimistic person accepts that life will throw up problems and setbacks, but feels that she can face them and survive them. She takes responsibility for the things that she has some control over, and doesn't blame herself for events which are not her fault.

Some people do seem to be genetically prone to being optimistic or pessimistic. However, even if your natural inclination is always to look on the dark side, you can develop a more optimistic attitude. Developing a calmer, more positive approach to life really will help you to manage your angry moments.

Find the good in situations

Use the reframing strategy which we discussed earlier. This will pull you up when you find you are slipping into a low mood and are unable to see the good in a situation. Reframe in order to:

- keep it in perspective;
- discover any good which might come out of something bad.

I'll never get a job

Charlotte has been applying for jobs, with no success so far. She has become anxious and tense about this, and is seeing herself as an absolute failure in the world of work. She says that the way she is going she will never get a job, and she is losing the will to keep sending out applications.

Charlotte could take a different angle on her situation. A positive reframing to keep things in perspective might be:

'I am not a failure, I just haven't found a job yet. Of course I will get one if I persevere with my applications. I know I am very employable. There is an employer out there who will want what I have to offer. What I have to do is to find this person.'

A positive reframing to discover the good in the situation might be:

'I am learning from this experience. I am discovering my strengths and weaknesses, and am developing qualities of perseverance and tenacity.'

Don't spend too much time with angry people

Listening to a good moan or rant can be enjoyable, particularly if the rant is expressed in a lively and entertaining way. There is a danger, though, in too much exposure to constant negativity. Anger and cynicism, even expressed as jokes, can rub off on you and affect your own outlook on life.

Don't spend too much time with people who bring you down

If you feel that being in the company of certain people leaves you feeling angry, scratchy, irritated or generally out of sorts, ask yourself:

- Why do I feel like this?
- Is this a situation I want to avoid or one I need to address?
- Do I need to continue to see this person?

Leah cuts contact

Leah and Libby each have young babies and, having met at the clinic during their pregnancies, are in the habit of a weekly meeting for a cup of coffee in one of the local places that easily accommodates prams and pushchairs. Leah used to look forward to this break, but recently has found that, no matter what mood she was in previously, she leaves their meeting feeling somehow down and ready to be annoyed at the slightest thing.

Leah realizes that Libby monopolizes their conversation with a series of moans about all aspects of her life – how tired she is, how no one understands the pressures of looking after small children, how she gave up a successful career and will never get back on that ladder, how their house is too small but they can't afford to move – on and on she goes, while Leah nods sympathetically and tries not to mind when all her attempts to widen the scope of their conversation are overridden by Libby's determination to focus on the negative. The effect of this

situation is to make Leah herself feel somehow disgruntled and dis-
satisfied, although she isn't, and she ends up frustrated that she has
to listen to all this stuff.

Leah could bring this up with Libby, but she decides that it isn't
worth it. She knows that Libby goes into moaning mode with everyone,
and Leah thinks that it is not worth the emotional energy required to
deal with this situation. Libby's is not a friendship that she wants to
cultivate.

The problem is solved by Leah deciding to be unable to make their
meetings. She feels much better now that she isn't exposed to that
regular burst of negativity.

In that situation, Leah's choice was comparatively easy. Often,
however, we are in the position of having to, or indeed wanting
to, spend time with people who bring us down – family members,
work colleagues, friends we are fond of although their company
tends to be depressing. In these cases you might need to choose a
strategy to help you to minimize the effect they have on you.

You could:

- Gently describe to the person the aspects of their behaviour that
  bring you down and describe the effect on you: 'I know a lot of
  your friends have had operations recently and that you like to
  talk about all the details but, you know, I don't enjoy that kind
  of thing. Can we talk about something else?'
- Distract the person by drawing their attention to something else
  every time they start the depressing stuff: 'Oh, sorry to interrupt,
  but look at that person over there'; 'Have you seen this memo?';
  'Did you hear that funny noise?' This strategy might break the
  flow and give you a chance to change the subject.
- Do something while they are talking, to dilute your attention –
  tidy up, start preparing dinner, load the dishwasher, tidy your
  handbag, look at your emails … This will protect you from
  the full onslaught and will let the person know that you aren't
  giving them your full attention.

Exercise 10.3: Dealing with negativity

Identify people in your life who have a negative effect on your mood.
Decide how you are going to deal with the situation.

Person	What they do or say	How I feel	What I can do

Don't bring yourself down

Don't dwell on the grim and tragic aspects of the news. You want to be aware of what is going on in the world, but ask yourself if it is doing you any good to fill your mind with the distressing details of, for example, horrific cases of murder or child abuse.

The power of laughter

Laugh as much as you can. You can't feel angry when you are laughing. Make a point of watching films and TV programmes that you find funny. Read articles and columns that always make you smile. If you have a favourite cartoon in a newspaper or magazine, cut out any that you particularly like and put them on the fridge or next to your computer, to give you a laugh whenever you see them.

Spend time with people who make you feel good

Make a point of spending time with people who raise your spirits and whose company you find interesting and stimulating. There may be people in your life who make you laugh, or whose positive outlook always has a good effect on you. Don't just leave their influence to chance – decide who these people are and plan the kind of contact you would like.

Exercise 10.4: Good company

Person	How they raise my spirits	Plan to contact

Spend time with people who help you

Develop a positive network of people who can help you to address and find solutions for problems and challenges. There may be someone who can act as your personal or business mentor or coach, or someone who offers you spiritual or emotional sustenance. Look for people who will offer you constructive criticism and feedback, as well.

Be ready to support and help others

Giving to others has reciprocal benefits – you feel good as well. Look for opportunities where you can make a difference to someone else, practically, emotionally, in whatever way is appropriate.

Be committed

Commitment is one of the characteristics of a resilient personality, one that is able to cope with challenge and turbulence and feels in control. It involves being actively engaged in what you do and finding contentment in your activities. Meeting life full on with a sense of purpose and direction demonstrates trust and optimism, and keeps your spirits buoyant.

Become more tolerant

The more we experience and understand people not like ourselves, the more tolerant and accepting we are likely to be. Our natural instinct is to seek out and spend time with people who are similar to us, but you could extend your comfort zone and encounter people who are different from you. Listening to and empathizing with someone who is of an older or younger generation, or someone with different values and beliefs, can widen your range of understanding and raise your tolerance levels so that negative responses are not so readily triggered.

Finding inner peace

Meditation

Meditation has been practised for thousands of years, and research continues to verify the physical and psychological benefits of this practice. The state of deep relaxation which meditation induces is an antidote to stress and can change your life significantly. Practitioners find that their tension disappears and that they develop a more positive, focused and tolerant approach to life. Their capacity for enjoyment is also increased, as is their ability to empathize with others.

There are various schools and types of meditation, but most of them are based on principles of relaxation, restfulness and stilling your mind. Meditation is really the opposite of what we do in our daily lives as we rush from activity to activity with our minds buzzing and teeming with thoughts, plans, emotions, desires, anxieties, fretfulness. When you meditate you are still alert and aware, but you make your mind become absolutely still and you exist just in the moment. You don't dream or worry about the future or think about the past.

Central to many forms of meditation is the idea that you focus on one single thing – it could be one word, or a sound, or a prayer, or an image. Other thoughts may float into your mind, but you let them float out again and return to your focus. Don't try to force anything; just let everything have its own pace.

You can explore the topic of meditation further and develop your own methods. Here is one exercise you might try:

- Sit in a quiet place, in a comfortable position.
- Close your eyes.
- Relax your body, working through each muscle group in turn until you feel loose and floppy.
- Breathe deeply and slowly.
- As you breathe in, hear your chosen word inside your head. Repeat it as you breathe out.

Try this for about five minutes at first. Twenty minutes a day will give you optimum results.

Meditation becomes more effective the more you practise it, so you could try to build sessions into your usual routine.

Visualization

This involves creating a picture in your head and bringing it to your mind when it's needed. It's a great way of moving yourself into a

calm and relaxed state, and as with meditation, the more you practise this technique the easier you will find it to access a peaceful
state of mind.

Make your own picture, one which works for you. Sit somewhere
quiet and solitary, and close your eyes. Conjure up a place which
brings about feelings of peace and well-being. Many people choose
images of nature, but the precise type of picture depends on what
appeals to you. It might be a sandy beach bathed in warm sunshine,
or a spring meadow carpeted with flowers, or a magnificent wild
mountain, or a garden with bees buzzing among the flowers and a
stream rippling ... You could try to create a place which involves
more than one of your senses. If you can hear the leaves rustling or
the stream tumbling down the mountainside, and if you can feel
the sun on your back or the grass beneath your feet, your picture
will be all the more vibrant in your consciousness. Your place might
be somewhere you know, somewhere you visited once or somewhere you visit often. It might even be a place that is part of your
everyday life, such as a room at home which fills you with peace
and calm.

Whatever image you are using, just having it ready and knowing
it is there for you to enter, any time you want to opt out for a few
minutes and let yourself relax, is in itself a calming thought.

Exercise 10.5: My plan for peaceful living

Work out your own individual plan for peaceful, anger-free living. Decide
what you will do on a regular basis to help you to stay calm and self-
controlled. Add your own ideas to the suggested categories if you wish.

	Every day	*Every month*	*Every year*
Emotional well-being			
Physical well-being			
Spiritual well-being			
Social well-being			

Useful addresses

British Association of Anger Management
Kingscote
East Grinstead
West Sussex RH19 4LG
Tel.: 0845 1300 286
Website: www.angermanage.co.uk

British Association for Counselling and Psychotherapy
BACP House
15 St John's Business Park
Lutterworth
Leics LE17 4HB
Tel.: 01455 883300
Website: www.bacp.co.uk

Drinkline
Tel.: 0800 917 8282 (24 hours a day, 7 days a week)

National Domestic Violence Helpline
Tel.: 0808 2000 247 (24 hours a day, 7 days a week)
Website: www.womensaid.org.uk

Relate
Central Office
Premier House
Carolina Court
Lakeside
Doncaster DN4 5RA
Tel.: 0300 100 1234 (8 a.m. to 10 p.m., Monday to Thursday; 8 a.m. to
6 p.m., Friday; 9 a.m. to 5 p.m., Saturday)
Website: www.relate.org.uk

Further reading

Fisher, Mike (2005), *Beating Anger*, Random House, London

Gentry, W. Doyle (2007), *Anger Management for Dummies*, Wiley, Chichester

Gottman, John (2000), *Seven Principles for Making Marriage Work*, Orion, London

Schiraldi, Glenn R. and Kerr, Melissa Hallmark (2002), *The Anger Management Sourcebook*, McGraw-Hill, New York

Thayer, Robert E. (1988), *The Origin of Everyday Moods*, Oxford University Press US, New York

Index

133